BREAKING THE AGE BARRIER

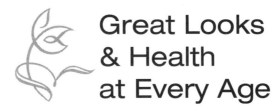

Great Looks
& Health
at Every Age

OLEDA BAKER

BREAKING THE AGE BARRIER

Great Looks
& Health
at Every Age

OLEDA BAKER

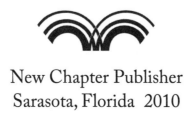

New Chapter Publisher

Sarasota, Florida 2010

Published by New Chapter Publisher

BREAKING THE AGE BARRIER
Great Looks & Health at Every Age

ISBN 978-0-9841745-9-1

New Chapter Publisher
1765 Ringling Blvd.
Suite 300
Sarasota, FL 34236
tel. 941-954-4690
www.newchapterpublisher.com

BREAKING THE AGE BARRIER
is distributed by Midpoint Trade Books

Printed in the United States of America

Cover design and layout by Shaw Creative
www.shawcreativegroup.com

DEDICATION

To my loving husband, Richard, who has been unbelievably supportive, not only with this book, but with everything I do.

To my son David.

To all women who want to look, feel and be younger all their lives...and know they can.

To my very talented editor, Chris Angermann, whose nonstop dedication to put out the best book possible has been invaluable.

ACKNOWLEDGMENTS

Writing this book involved a large number of people whose influence and advice have been significant over time. I thank them all for their unwavering support.

Here I would just like to mention:

My father, who led the way to my thinking "prevention."

My mother, who taught me by example the value of taking care of my looks.

My 4 stepdaughters, Kathy, Daryl, Sue and Ann, who have been an inspiration, each in her own unique way.

My longtime friend and associate, Linda Haun, whose sage advice has been invaluable.

My dearest friend of 45 years, Vernice Gabriel, who has encouraged me through all trials and tribulations.

At New Chapter Publisher, Piero Rivolta, who recognized the importance of this book; my editor, Chris Angermann and his wife Susan; Inna Yakubova, who helped with the editing, and Vanessa Houston, who put the finishing touches on the book.

Seven people who outsmarted their genes and were kind enough to share with me how they did it: Howard Ackerman, Lynn Baron, Herbert Kanter, David Kazarian, Susan Scholsohn, Joan and Robert Wolff. Their powerful stories can be found at www.oleda.com.

And finally, a toast to my personal lady friends, who know that "girlfriend time" is so valuable for our health and well-being—thanks, girls!

Contents

NABIL K. ABOUKHAIR, MD PA
Gynecology & Infertility

I have been Oleda Baker's physician since 1994 and have full access to her files. Over the past 15 years, in all her annual exams and tests, such as cholesterol, blood pressure, and all others typically performed, I can give a firsthand account of her physical condition and medical well-being. Oleda has consistently scored as would a healthy person at least 25 years younger than her actual age of 75.

She is in excellent physical condition and without any chronic or acute ailments. Other than a strictly monitored hormone replacement therapy treatment, I do not prescribe for Oleda any medications to be taken on a regular basis. At every annual exam, Oleda continues to amaze me with her excellent blood pressure, low cholesterol and other parameters, such as optimum weight, physical strength and bone density. Oleda has the bone density of a woman in her 20s. I am proud to be Oleda Baker's physician, for she is an excellent example of how a woman should maintain her physical health and remain ever youthful.

12-29-09

Nabil Aboukair, MD PA

I recently examined Ms. Baker for any signs of a facelift. After inspecting her scalp, ears and other areas where surgical scars may be present indicating a surgical facelift...there was no evidence of any surgical scars noted.

Dr. Karen R. Tobman
Board Certified in Podiatric Medicine and Orthopedics
Boca Raton, Florida

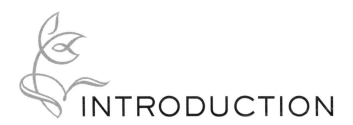

INTRODUCTION

The picture of me on the cover of this book was taken when I was 75 years old. Of course, I have makeup on and the photographer used professional lighting, but absolutely no retouching or Photoshop work of any kind was done. I have never had a facelift, although I did have the skin around my eyes tightened many years ago, because I did a lot of close-up "beauty" ads and felt it would benefit my career as a model. As the letter on the opposite page points out, my physician certifies that for the past 15 years, my annual exams and tests have consistently shown that I have the body and health of someone at least 25 years younger than me.

Perhaps you're thinking, "It must be in her DNA. How could a 75-year-old look that way without having great genes?" So let me tell you what my dear, loving brother Harry has allowed me to say about him: Harry, who is three years my junior, weighs 345 pounds and is the first to admit that his health is not good. He has had heart surgery and a knee replacement. He's in constant pain from arthritis, especially in his hips and back, and he's tired all the time. Having had the same mother and father, we come from the same gene pool. The difference between Harry and me has been our lifestyles…and he agrees.

Of course, the genes you inherited are very important to your health, but they are not as influential as you might believe. A long-term study of identical twins[1,2] concluded that 70% of the aging process is due to lifestyle and environment, and only 30% is the result of DNA.

By the way, both of my parents were overweight at one point, and my father, at age 40, was in poor health until he took charge of his well-being…which is how my interest in anti-aging began. I was 14 at the time. I saw how my father managed to change his life on his own, and I never forgot it.

But, let's talk about you. If you want to look, feel and be younger for the rest of your life, I can help you achieve that goal, just as I have done for myself. The art of ageless beauty and vibrant health is something that I have studied and tested all my life. I have walked the walk. I have lived my life searching for what works, and along the way I've learned what does not work. You will find that the advice in this book is "real" and simple to follow.

Many women (and men) do not know the variety of choices available today that can keep them looking and feeling more youthful and vital longer in life. Some think they can start later, and end up waiting until it's too late to make the necessary changes in their lifestyle. Others just accept their "fate," or think it's not important. Mother Nature works against us every day of our lives…some people just stand by and let her do it…don't be one of them.

A few years ago, turning 50, once thought of as old, became "a new beginning." But, hold it…have you noticed what's happening today to those hitting 70? Look around you: for many, 70 is becoming "middle age," and they are having the time of their healthy lives. Some even start another career and do things their parents never dreamed of doing at 60! This book tells you how to achieve your own new beginning…all the way to your own vivacious older years.

> I WISH I COULD GET EVERYONE TO THINK ABOUT THEIR LONGEVITY AND THE IMPACT THAT DAY-TO-DAY BEHAVIOR HAS, NOT ONLY ON HOW LONG YOU WILL LIVE, BUT HOW WELL YOU CAN LIVE THOSE EXTENDED YEARS.

Many of my "secrets" are not new. You may even recognize some of them from my other books or from my website—tried-and-true anti-aging methods the effectiveness of which has been verified over the course of many years. What is different and unique about this book is the way it puts them all together as a complete guide and program, both in detail and overall approach, combining internal and external practices.

I believe that vibrant aging can only be achieved if you treat the inside and outside of your entire body at the same time. For example, if you eat the wrong foods and lack good nutrition, you can lather on all the creams and lotions in the world, and your skin will still begin to show signs of aging much sooner than you think. On the other hand, you can eat all the right foods, but neglect proper treatment of the surface of your skin and the collagen beneath it, and you will still not have the long-term beautiful skin you deserve.

You need to think in terms of the whole body—head to toe, inside and out—and work on it all at the same time. It's much easier and faster than tackling one "piece" at a time. Once you get comfortable with a routine, each "piece" helps other "pieces," and the crossovers speed up the process. It's not a magic pill or an overnight fix, however.

Many people have allowed their good looks, energy and health to deteriorate for many years. If your beauty and body are badly out of shape and you want to achieve serious success with this book, you need to set a realistic time frame of up to one year to see results. That might seem like a long time in today's fast-paced world. Most of us are spoiled because of the electronic age we live in; we want results now. But good health and beauty for life can't be achieved with an "instant fix" approach. There are no shortcuts,

The reason it might take a year is that some areas of your body, such as bone cells, take that long to regenerate. Others, like soft tissue cells, take less time to improve. For some of you, it may only take 2 or 3 months…but you'll have to read this book to find out if you are one of them! The good news is that you can help prevent your own aging, and even help reverse it, more than ever before.

Your interest in your health and beauty is coming exactly at the right time. Never before has scientific and medical research made it so easy to stay young and vital as we grow older—to remain beautiful and glamorous throughout our whole lives. If 70 is becoming our middle age, we should be able to live beyond 100 years, as modern medicine suggests, perhaps even as long as 125! You don't want to live to be a feeble 125, you say? How about just a very healthy, beautiful 95-year-old?

Even with all the advances in science and medical research, none of us can assume that a long, healthy life span is a given. Each of us must assume the day-to-day responsibility that ensures a flexible, healthy body with lots of energy, youthful skin and hair, and the ability to help prevent illness. Medical breakthroughs, past and future, are only part of the journey toward your very own long, healthy, beautiful life. You must step up and help yourself. No one else can or will do it for you.

Let's begin…

Love,

Oleda

PART 1: OUTSIDE

Mother Nature can't help you,
and Father Time is not on your side.

What's the first thing you notice when you meet a person for the first time? Is it the eyes, the shape, the hair, or the skin? Many people say it's the skin. So, the appearance of your skin is likely an important factor in determining how people react to you in that initial instant. Other things, like your personality, take over from there, but why not start strong with the first look?

Fifty years ago, I went to New York City, intent on becoming a high fashion model. I was 26, which was considered "old" for a model in those days. Somehow, at the famous Ford Model Agency, I got through the initial interviews, and the staff sent me in to meet Eileen Ford herself. To my surprise and delight, she invited me to join her agency and gave me a list of places to go to the next day. Eileen wasn't put off by my age. She said, "You look 19, you are 19!" I am convinced to this day that, besides being slim—the number one job requirement—what impressed her most was the youthful condition of my skin, which I had taken exceptional care of.

Before I left for New York, a friend in Miami who knew Natalie Paine, owner of Ford's rival model agency, Plaza Five, had given me a package to deliver to her as a personal gift. After my meeting with Eileen Ford, I stopped at Plaza Five unannounced to drop off the present. Much to my surprise, I was ushered into Natalie's office. When she asked what I was doing in New York and I told her about my visit with Eileen Ford, she said, "Well, dear, Eileen wants you, and I want you, too."

I liked Natalie Paine. She was very sweet—the complete opposite of Eileen Ford, who was known for her toughness—and I decided to join Plaza Five. Now, a few of Natalie's models were 10 years younger than me, so here again, I attribute her initial positive impressions of me to the appearance of my skin and my ability to "put my best face forward."

Later on, when Wilhelmina, one of Ford's top models, left and started her own agency, she invited me to join her, and I did. Those were spectacular times. I was with Wilhelmina Models until age 38 when I started my own business, Oleda and Company, Inc., developing and marketing beauty, health and anti-aging products. Had I not kept my skin at its best, I imagine I would probably have taken a very different road in life.

CHAPTER 1

SKIN CARE FOR LIFELONG HEALTH AND BEAUTY

*It's not the kind of skin you were born with that matters
—it's what you do to the skin you were born with.*

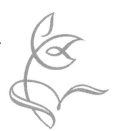

The skin of the hands, face and neck ages fastest because it is exposed to the environment every day. Wind, sun, pollution, air conditioning and wintertime heating all take their toll. But there are other factors as well, such as poor circulation, improper nutrition, and dryness.

Treating the surface is only the beginning for retaining beautiful, youthful skin for life. The cells beneath it, the supporting muscles, the bones, nutritional intake and general health all interact, affecting the beauty and aging of your skin. Creams and lotions are very important in helping to retain its youthful look, but it will take more—much more—than that.

For lifelong, youthful, beautiful-looking skin, there are specific things you must do—and must not do. If you are young and think, "I don't need to start at my age," you are missing the boat. Without proactive treatment the surface of the skin begins degenerating at about age 20, even though the signs are not yet visible.

There is a protein produced in the dermis—the sub-surface layer of the skin that gives it strength and resilience. It is called collagen and it can begin to breakdown and harden even early in life, depending on the degree of bad habits. It may take a few years for the damage to show up, but collagen breakdown leads to premature small lines and wrinkles, which result in other aging skin problems as well. Many baby boomers are just now realizing that abusing their skin when they were young has left its mark, and they are scrambling to try to correct it now.

The good news is that no matter how old you are, it is not too late, but the earlier you begin caring for your skin, the easier it will be in the long run.

Fifty years ago during my early days as a model, I learned from my more experienced colleagues how to keep my skin flawless. Soon I became engrossed, perhaps even a little obsessed, with figuring out how to preserve and protect my youthful, healthy skin for the rest of my life. Since my skin is ultra dry, I know how shriveled it would look today if I had not done that, and then put what I learned into practice…every day.

As you know, the skin is your largest organ, wrapping your entire body. It has many daily "chores" besides acting as a barrier against damage from external and internal forces. It helps regulate heat and moisture evaporation, and provides you with a sense of touch. Every day, you lose 30,000 or 40,000 dead cells that flake off the surface. Those old cells became tough and strong as they protected your body. Meanwhile, the epidermis constantly makes new cells that rise to the surface to replace the old ones.

That's why your diet is so important to the health of all your cells, including those of your skin. If you don't eat the right foods, your cells will not regenerate as efficiently. Put too many of the wrong foods in your mouth, and your skin will show it. So you see, it's really in your hands!

The principles and practices in this chapter pertain to everybody, whether you were born with skin of color as in Africa and Asia, or you came into the world with the fair skin of people with a Northern European background. All skin can be dry, normal or oily, as the case may be. And, while skin of color contains more of the pigment melanin, which determines color tone and guards somewhat against the sun's rays, thus resulting in fewer wrinkles and crow's-feet, it still needs protection and treatment. The sun can darken skin of color and once that occurs, it can take years to get it back to normal.

In general, a woman's skin is thinner than a man's, thus more susceptible to the sun's rays, but that doesn't mean that men should be any less careful.

Be especially sure to protect children. Their skin is young and tender, and the sun's rays can cause serious problems more quickly. Just one serious sunburn in a young child can be enough to cause serious damage for life.

Daily Needs for Your Skin Type

Dry Skin

Cells sloughing off the body's surface too quickly interferes with the skin's ability to retain moisture, resulting in dry skin. While moisturizing creams and lotions are needed for all skin types, they are especially necessary for dry skin and have to be applied more frequently throughout the day.

If your skin is dry and happens to be the kind of skin you were born with, you simply need to learn to compensate for it (as I have). But if it is caused by your environment—such as indoor heating during the winter—or by a deficiency in the proper nutrients, you might consider changing your surroundings or diet. Dry skin also loses its moisture through dehydration and evaporation from exposure to sun, wind and cold air, so you'll need to compensate for Mother Nature.

More than 50% of women have dry skin, and they should never use soap and water to remove their makeup. This sucks moisture from the pores, exacerbating the problem. There are makeup-removing creams and lotions available for this purpose that leave the skin moist. If you are a person who doesn't feel cleansed without using water on your face, okay. After you use a cream or lotion makeup remover, rinse with cool water…but then be sure to apply plenty of moisturizing cream afterwards.

Note: *Make sure you apply a rich night cream before you go to sleep.*

Normal Skin

Just because your skin is normal—that is to say, well-balanced with oils and moisture—that doesn't mean you can neglect it. If you do, it won't stay normal for long. It's best to follow most of the instructions here that apply to dry skin. Cleanse with a cream or lotion to keep moisture in. Use a rich moisturizer cream after cleansing. Apply a rich night cream before you go to sleep.

Oily Skin

Proper cleansing is vital in order to keep the pores unclogged and to help minimize an oily look and greasy feel. Use lightweight cleansing products, not heavy creams. After cleansing use a toner astringent to remove any residual oils or bacteria that might be left on the skin's surface or in the pores. Scrubs with granules are great for oily skin. Always use a light moisturizing cream after cleansing; never leave your skin feeling taut or dry. Even oily skin needs to be protected and nourished throughout the day.

Some parts of your face might have oily skin, while others are dry or normal. If the oily parts are a serious problem, they can be cleansed more frequently than the dry sections. You can also dab the oily spots with a tissue or an oil-blotting powder during the day. Use a toner astringent in the morning and at night before applying makeup and before retiring to bed after cleansing. It's best to follow both the dry skin and oily skin routines as needed. Carry tissues with you to occasionally pat or press down on the spots. This removes the oils without adding extra powder.

SPECIAL NEEDS FOR AFRICAN-AMERICAN SKIN

In general, African-American skin requires no different care than fair skin. Skin is skin. However, there are some specific differences that may require special attention. For example, the higher melanin content of black skin provides some natural protection from the ravages of aging caused by the ultraviolet rays of the sun. Make no mistake, however: If you are dark-skinned, you must still protect yourself from the sun. You are still subject to both skin cancer—although 20 times less likely to get it—and deepening in color (an unprotected black face can become a lot darker than protected parts of the body).

FLESH MOLES

Raised brown or black dark spots that appear mostly on the cheeks, flesh moles occur most frequently in black women, and tend to be hereditary. A variant of a condition called seborrheic keratosis, they are not cancerous, but some people may decide to have them removed for cosmetic reasons. Consistent use of sunscreen can prevent them from becoming darker and increasing in size.

VITILIGO

This condition manifests itself in the form of irregular white splotches on the face, hands and chest, although they may occur elsewhere on the body as well. Sometimes, the white patches can grow larger until they blend together and form larger areas of colorless skin. Vitiligo is the result of damaged pigment. While scientists suspect that it is caused by problems with the auto-immune system, nobody knows for sure; there is some evidence that it may be hereditary.

There are a number of different treatments for vitiligo, none of them perfect. Let your dermatologist determine which is best, depending on the extent of the condition. The most common treatment is called PUVA, a combination of a photosensitizing agent and ultraviolet light. Other methods include cortisone creams or laser treatment and even skin grafting.

Flaky Skin

If you're black and have dry, flaky skin, you have probably noticed that it has a gray, ashy color. Using makeup to hide the problem may make it worse. It's a vicious circle. The only way to correct this condition is to use moisturizers liberally and frequently. Over-the-counter products are fine, but I would suggest you find one that has aloe vera as one of the primary ingredients.

Keloids

Keloids are the excess growth of scar tissue where an injury to the skin has healed. Lumpy or ridged, they cover the site of a wound. They usually occur on the chest, back, arms or earlobes. Treatments include cortisone injections, silicone gels, surgery, laser treatment, liquid nitrogen and radiation; however, once removed, they often return, sometimes larger than before.

The Danger of Sun Exposure

The sun, doctors agree, is the most powerful aging agent of skin, resulting in more wrinkles than any other cause, including smoking. And it is cumulative. The more exposure to the sun over the years, the more deep wrinkles you will have. The more "burns" you sustain, the faster your skin will age and the greater the likelihood that you will develop skin cancer. It's amazing that, despite all the medical warnings, incidents of skin cancer increase each year.

I was very lucky when I was young. The hot sun on my skin actually "hurt." I couldn't take it, so I protected it with hats and long sleeves. I have never "baked" in the sun and have never suffered sunburn.

The trouble is that the damage is invisible for some time until all of a sudden we notice the change in our skin and blame the last few times we were in the sun. But it starts years earlier when collagen begins hardening under the surface of the skin.

Years ago it was thought that soaking up the rays of the sun was actually healthy. We now know how wrong that was, yet so many of us still don't pay attention to it; we want that fashionable, tanned skin. Thank you, Coco Chanel for starting an unhealthy trend more than 70 years ago! But the sun's ultraviolet rays, the penetrating ones that produce a tan for Caucasians and darken black skin, also cause the skin to burn, shrivel up (wrinkle) and, of course, develop skin cancer.

As for the health benefits of sunshine, they are overrated. Did you know that just 10 minutes of sun three days a week on a small part of your body will provide you with the recommended requirement of vitamin D?

It is estimated that about one-third of adults in the U.S. will suffer bad sunburn at least once. UV rays are more intense in the summer, at high altitudes and closer to the equator. But the sun's harmful effects are also increased by wind and reflections from water, sand and snow.

No matter how much exposure to the sun you have suffered, it's never too late to begin protecting yourself.

- Most important: Use a sunblock or sunscreen with an SPF (Sun Protection Factor) of at least 15. But SPF numbers are the result of laboratory tests performed under controlled conditions. People often don't apply as much sunscreen as was done in the lab, reducing its effectiveness. In addition, swimming, toweling or wiping a portion of the body for any reason removes the sunscreen. So use it liberally and reapply frequently. If you want to be completely safe, use a total sunblock. It doesn't look pretty—as you know, it's thicker and usually white in color—but it works.

- Wear a wide-brimmed hat that shades the back and sides of your neck, too.

> MOST PEOPLE THINK THAT A HIGHER SPF NUMBER MEANS A SUNSCREEN PROVIDES GREATER PROTECTION. THEY DON'T REALIZE THAT THE SPF NUMBERS REPRESENT THE LENGTH OF TIME OF PROTECTION. A SUNSCREEN WITH AN SPF OF 15 SAFEGUARDS AGAINST SOLAR RAYS 15 TIMES LONGER THAN IF NO SUNSCREEN WERE USED. A SUNSCREEN WITH AN SPF OF 30 OR HIGHER, OFFERS NO STRONGER PROTECTION THAN SPF No.15, BUT, THEORETICALLY, PREVENTS YOUR SKIN FROM BURNING 30 TIMES LONGER THAN IT WOULD WITHOUT SUNSCREEN, OR TWICE AS LONG AS SPF No.15.

- Wear protective clothing for the occasion.

- If possible, schedule outdoor activities before 10 a.m. or after 3 p.m. when ultraviolet rays are less intense.

- Be especially careful during the summer when UV exposure is as much as 100 times greater than in winter. The ozone layer above North America is thinnest in late summer/early fall.

- Be careful at higher altitudes, whether you live there or are just visiting. For every 1000-foot increase in elevation, UV exposure increases an average of 7%.

Avoid tanning beds. A recent scientific study determined that people who use tanning devices were 1.5 to 2.5 times more likely to develop common kinds of skin cancer than people who did not use them.[3] The ultraviolet radiation from tanning beds causes aging and skin cancer, just as the sun does.

If you want to appear tanned, use a good quality indoor overnight sunless tanning lotion. There are several over-the-counter types to choose from. I recommend wearing gloves and applying the lotion with a soft, rounded sponge. If you're not using gloves, make sure to wash your hands with warm soapy water immediately afterwards. To prevent unevenness, streaks or splotches, follow these rules.

- Exfoliate your skin first. You can utilize a rough washcloth; a loofah is good, too. This gets rid of the dry, scaly skin that is about to "flake off" anyway, helps the product to go on evenly and ensures longer wear. Give extra attention to exfoliating the areas where dead skin accumulates, such as knees, elbows, ankles, hands and feet.

- Take a shower or bath to remove all oil from your skin, as the active ingredient in the tanning lotion clings best to a freshly buffed, non-oily surface.

- After you've dried off, apply the lotion with long firm full strokes. Then rub it in with a circular motion so it blends into the skin better and is streak-free.

- Always start from your lower body and work your way up. This helps to avoid the creases and smudges that develop when you bend over to apply the lotion. First cover the areas between your ankles and knees. Then apply what remains to your feet, ankles and knees, which do not need as much tanner.

- To keep knees from soaking up too much tanner, either wipe off any excess lotion right away, or apply moisturizer and then wipe it off.

- After covering the rest of the body, wipe any excess from the elbows.

- Wait about 8 hours before moisturizing the skin or working out, which will cause you to perspire.

If you have dark spots on your skin you don't want to tan, remove the tanning lotion by lightly twirling a moistened Q-tip on the dark spot, making sure not to go beyond its perimeter. If you want a darker tan, repeat this process the next day.

DEALING WITH DRYNESS IN WINTER

The dry, cold winter months can be especially hard on skin, as chapped lips make all too clear. So it's easy to feel like a failure when you can't keep your skin moist. (After all, you can't very well rub Chapstick all over your body.) Failing year after year, however, will cause permanent premature aging of the skin. It's frustrating and you might begin to think it's something you must accept.

Wrong! Here's what to do to have moist, soft skin all winter long.

Adjust your bathing habits. Take shorter tub baths or showers and use tepid water. If you feel comfortable doing so, alternate the way you "bathe" by applying soap only to your armpits, bottom, hands and feet every other time. Dry off gently, patting the skin dry in order to retain as much natural moisture as possible. Bathing does not contribute to the skin's dryness, as long as you limit the use of soap and lubricate your skin immediately afterwards. After each bath or shower, replace lost moisture with a good body lotion. An aloe vera based body lotion is best. If you are prone to dry spots throughout the day, keep the body lotion handy and apply it in the dry areas again.

Note: For serious dry skin patches on the body, try an over-the-counter hydrocortisone cream.

If your skin itches, it may be because of dry air causing moisture in the top layer of the skin to evaporate quickly. Rub a rich cream on these spots, even an ointment-like cream. You'll feel relief in a few minutes.

Do you have flaking skin? During winter, there can be literally thousands of dry skin cells, invisible to the eye, that can clump together with oil, forming flakes that are ready to be sloughed off the surface. Lightly remove them with a rough washcloth or a loofah, and apply a rich cream immediately, gently rubbing it into the skin.

Don't forget that what you eat and drink has a lot to do with the moisture level in your body, including your skin and hair. Drink plenty of water and juice every day. Dry skin can also be compensated for by a good, nutritious, balanced diet.

SCARS AND STRETCH MARKS

I often get asked what to do about scars and stretch marks: Can you really get rid of them? Now don't fault me for this, but the answer is yes, no, maybe and sometimes, it depends on! I used to believe they were here to stay, but there are new products and new procedures that give hope for some—not all—types of scars and stretch marks.

Note: If you have a new scar, keep it out of the sun, apply sunscreen to it, and try to keep it moist with vitamin E cream while it is healing.

There are several brands of scar sheets sold over the counter now in drugstores and supermarkets. These adhesive patches contain silicone, which can soften scars. They work best on raised (hypertrophic) scars, and should not be used until the wound closes and the scar heals. Silicone patches must be worn for at least 8 weeks to get results. There are also topical gels that may help reduce such scars. Some of the brand names are Band-Aid, Neosporin and Mederma.

Flat (normotrophic) scars that are the same height as the surrounding normal skin are the most difficult to get rid of. Such blemishes can sometimes be improved on by a medical doctor specializing in dermatology, with new procedures available, such as laser resurfacing.

Depressed (hypotrophic or atrophic) scars can be raised by a dermatologist or registered nurse under a doctor's supervision by injecting collagen beneath them.

Unfortunately, there is less hope for stretch marks. They generally appear because of rapid weight gain, whether during pregnancy or for other reasons. Stretch marks can even be found in children who have become rapidly obese. Applying lotions, creams and ointments can help a little in some cases, especially if the extra weight was not put on too quickly. You should know that these marks sometimes can disappear or lessen after the cause of the skin stretching is gone.

SPECIAL SHAVING TIPS FOR WOMEN

There is one thing common to men that they can teach us women how to do better. Here's what I learned from my husband, Richard, on how to get the best, safest shave on my legs, underarms and bikini line.

- Make sure the blade in your razor is not dull. If you're in doubt, change it. There is really no difference in the quality of the shave when using a so-called, "women's razor," only the size, weight and balance of the razor. The blades that do the job are the same.

- Soften the hair; the best softener is water. So make sure you shave during or after a bath or shower, when the hair is moist. Dry hair is more difficult to cut, dulls a razor and greatly contributes to razor burn.

- Use a shave gel. There's a reason most men do so, rather than just relying on soap. The secret to a good smooth shave is moisture retention. Shave gel is designed to keep the hair and skin moist throughout the shave and to allow the razor to slide over the skin with less friction.

- Don't shave over skin eruptions. Go around them. You'll only open them up and make them worse.

- Don't be afraid to shave against the direction the hair is growing—against the grain, as it were. You can't get a close shave otherwise and will have to do it more frequently.

- Don't press down with the razor. Use a slow, light touch and, if necessary, more frequent strokes.

- Above all, don't rush. Shave s-l-o-w-l-y. The slower the shave, the better the shave.

- Use a moisturizer afterward. You have just attacked your skin and traumatized it by actually removing a layer of its cells. You need a good moisturizer and conditioner to revive it and keep it supple.

NUTRITION FOR GREAT SKIN

Glowing, vibrant and youthful-looking skin requires more than just creams and lotions. The foods you eat to feed the skin from the inside are just as important. It's never too late to change premature aging of the skin because of vitamin or nutrient deficiency. Your "building block cells" under the skin can change as you change your habits.

Special vitamins, minerals and herbs can help produce younger-looking, healthier skin. Your skin contains millions of cells, specialized nerve endings, numerous oil and sweat glands, hair follicles and blood vessels. The latter carry nourishment to this complex structure and directly affect the health, beauty and aging of your skin. Proper nutrition speeds up the blood flow, resulting in a richer source of "food" being carried to all three layers of skin—epidermis, dermis and the subcutaneous.

VITAMIN A is needed to prevent dryness and maintain elasticity.
Good sources: Meat, milk, cheese, eggs, spinach, carrots, squash and broccoli.

VITAMIN C keeps skin well-toned.
Good sources: Broccoli, kale, cabbage, strawberries and cantaloupe.

VITAMIN E restores moisture to the skin and slows down the aging of skin cells.
Good sources: Vegetable oil, green leafy vegetables and nuts.

As the years pass, you need more and more nutrition for your skin to remain in good shape. Present day trends in over-processed foods and fast foods make it more difficult to get all the nutrition we need just from the food we eat. I am a great believer in supplements (more on this in Chapter 6: Foods, Vitamins and Supplements).

HYDRATION/NATURAL CLEANSING

Good hydration plays an important role in keeping your skin looking healthy and youthful. This means drinking pure, clean water—not soda. It's difficult to drink the ideal amount—eight 8-ounce glasses of water a day—so I cheat a little. I take a small bite or 2 of a salty cracker, which helps me drink a lot more.

As we sleep at night our metabolism slows down, allowing our liver and kidneys to cleanse our bodies more efficiently. Once toxins are excreted, the skin looks much cleaner. When this process doesn't happen, because we don't sleep well, for example, our bodies continue to send blood to the major organs, not to the skin where it is needed. This results in fluids accumulating in the skin, especially around the eyes, and leads to that puffy-eyed look no one wants.

The best time to replenish the moisture the skin loses during the day, due to sun, wind and pollution, is while you're sleeping. When your metabolism slows, the cells are at rest and most available to absorb moisturizers. This is also a good reason to take a 15-minute nap during the day, if you can. Even if you just lie on the couch and allow every muscle in your body to relax with your eyes closed.

AFTERTHOUGHTS

Your body's largest organ encases you from head to toe, some 2,000 square inches on average; you should be comfortable showing off as much of it as you wish…or dare.

I'm still doing occasional modeling for my company. Recently we did a shoot, updating photographs of me for our website and catalog. I'm always anxious to see how the photos turn out, since I will not allow retouching of any kind. I'm pleased to say that they turned out well. I even dared to be photographed in a bikini…oh boy!

CHAPTER 2

HOW TO PUT YOUR BEST FACE FORWARD

*Great skin requires more
than just treating the surface.*

In this chapter, we will address all the things necessary to put your best face forward adding to what we covered in the previous discussion about how to treat your skin.

OK, now that you're doing all the right things, moisturizing your skin day and night, eating right and avoiding the sun, do you think that's it? Well, my friend, as you will see in this chapter, the answer to that question is, no, there's more. Now you need to preserve your skin's health and maintain its glow by using the techniques I've devised for myself, things that have helped me to keep my youthful-looking skin until now at age 75 and, trust me, going forward into my octogenarian years.

I would like to show you how to maintain long-term beauty with special facial exercises designed to keep your blood flow moving faster, nourishing the under layers of your skin and stimulating your collagen. Yes, you may have heard that facial exercises hurt the skin more than they help...and they will—if not done correctly. I've been doing these exercises for years.

Proper cleansing is very important for the health and refinement of the skin. You will learn in this chapter how to give yourself a mini facelift while cleansing your face. You will discover how to keep a more youthful neck and how to take care of that thin, sensitive skin around the eyes. What about hormones…can your skin use some? I discuss why and how to keep your "facial bones" stronger for tighter skin with fewer wrinkles. If you're contemplating professional treatment, look here for advice.

FACE-SAVING, FACE-LIFTING EXERCISES

Just a few minutes of easy exercises every day after cleansing and moisturizing can do wonders for your face by strengthening the muscles and increasing blood circulation. Along with creams and lotions, I credit these exercises for helping with my youthful-looking skin.

Building up your facial muscles is a slow, gradual process, so don't be discouraged if you don't see any results after the first few weeks. These exercises have a cumulative effect. It will take time, but, believe me, they're worth it!

I recommend that you do them once a day. However, if you find it difficult to keep to a daily routine, rest assured that you'll get good results with as little as three times a week.

You only need to do the exercises that apply to you.

To help smooth out crow's-feet and firm up droopy eyelids

- Close your eyes and squeeze the lids tightly for a slow count of three. Open and relax. Repeat for a total of 4 times.

- Place the fingertips of your left hand below the bottom lashes of your left eye, and the fingertips of your right hand below the bottom lashes of your right eye, gently. Don't press. Very slowly use your under eye muscles to try to close your eyes by moving the lower lids upward, taking special care not to wrinkle your forehead. Lift both lids as high as you can. Relax. Repeat for a total of 6 lifts.

To firm and lift cheeks and contour the sides of your face

- Place your finger vertically across the center of your mouth. Now, attempt to blow that finger away for a slow count of 10. The harder you blow, the harder your finger should resist. Relax, and then repeat 5 times. This helps keep cheeks firm and young-looking, and discourages the vertical "parentheses" lines that form from the nose to the corners of the mouth.

- Pull the muscles of your mouth outward without parting your lips. Use your muscles only, not your fingers! Hold for a count of 5, and then relax. Repeat 5 times.

To tone around the lips and lessen furrows between mouth and chin

- Say the word "church." Say it slowly and exaggerate the "ch" sound, so the peaks of your upper lip curl up. Try to make both your lips become rounder and fuller. Do that 12 times.

- With lips closed, fill the cheeks with air. When you reach the fullest point, hold for a count of 5. Relax, and then repeat 5 times.

To help rescue a double chin and tighten up jowls

- Stick your bottom lip out as far as it will go. Really pout! Hold for a slow count of 3. Relax. Repeat 5 times.

- Curl your tongue backward and press it against the roof of your mouth. Press hard, and then relax. Do this 6 times.

To help tighten and smooth horizontal lines and loose skin

- Stick out your tongue as far as it can go, then try to curl the tip upward. Unless you're Gene Simmons of Kiss, you probably won't be able to see it, but you'll get a wonderful tightening in the center of your neck. Repeat 10 times. To see how effective this exercise really is, bare your shoulders and look in the mirror. You'll see your neck muscles flex.

- Here's what I consider the best overall neck exercise: the Mona Lisa. Start to smile and stop in mid-smile, without parting your lips. Try to force the corners of your mouth upward, but don't let them rise. Repeat 12 times. Again, checking in the mirror will help you do it right.

When you have finished your exercises, lie down on your back with your head lower than the rest of your body. Relax for about 10 minutes.

This will encourage blood to rush to your head, feeding the outer layers of the skin, improving its texture and permeating it with the natural oils and moisture that will help prevent lines and wrinkles from forming. As a bonus, increased blood circulation to the head strengthens the roots of your hair. If you feel at all dizzy, sit up immediately.

"MINI FACELIFT" CLEANSING ROUTINE

Gently massaging the face and neck is a must for ageless skin. All of the body's cells should be stimulated, and the skin is no exception. For about 35 years I have given myself a quick "mini facelift" every night and in the morning as I cleanse my face and neck.

Many women avoid massaging their facial skin, fearful of permanently stretching it. However, my routine does not do that. Instead, it stimulates blood circulation and helps firm up the collagen under the skin, keeping it youthful, which in turn feeds more healthy nutrients to the dermis.

> IT TAKES ABOUT 3 MINUTES, AND YOU HAVE TO CLEANSE YOUR FACE ANYWAY!

The principal reason why massaging the face and neck is so beneficial can be found in the skin's own chemistry. As the skin's temperature rises, oil (sebum) is released, helping to clean out blackheads and clogged and enlarged pores, and leaving the skin cleaner, more radiant and glowing. This is why I call it a "Mini Facelift."

Step One: Cleanse your face and neck with your favorite makeup remover in an upward and outward motion. Use tissues or cloth until all makeup is gone. I go through as many tissues as I need, doubling them up for firmness. Do not pull down on the skin, use an up and out motion without stretching it. "Moving" the skin is fine…just don't force it.

Step Two: At this point, you might think your skin is clean, but it probably isn't. You need to be sure there's no trace of makeup left. Any impurities left in the pores will block the full benefit of a night cream or any other treatment you apply before going to bed. (You *are* putting something on your skin before you go to bed, aren't you!!?) To remove any such residue, use a washcloth and an astringent. The washcloth should be thin because you'll use less astringent/toner, yet get the job done. You can obtain inexpensive ones at a supermarket or discount store (I buy them by the bagful and reuse them after a turn in the washing machine).

Dampen a spot on the cloth with the astringent and gently rub it all over your face and neck—again using an upward and outward motion. You might

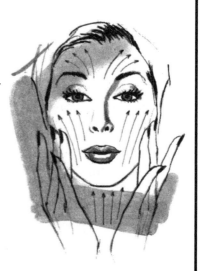

TWO VERY IMPORTANT RULES:

1. BE SURE YOU HAVE CLEANSED YOUR SKIN AND APPLIED CREAM TO YOUR FACE AND NECK AHEAD OF TIME. FACIAL EXERCISES DONE WHEN THE SKIN IS DRY MAY ACTUALLY HELP AGE IT. BUT DON'T ALLOW THE SKIN TO BE "SLIPPERY" AS YOU WILL NOT HAVE THE SAME RESULTS IF YOUR FINGERS JUST SLIDE LIGHTLY OVER THE SKIN SURFACE.

2. USE A FIRM HAND, BUT NEVER PULL THE SKIN IN A DOWNWARD DIRECTION, ONLY UPWARD AND OUTWARD. IF YOUR FACE STARTS TO TINGLE, THAT'S PROOF THAT YOU ARE STIMULATING AND FIRMING. (BY THE WAY, MEN WILL BENEFIT FROM THESE EXERCISES, TOO!)

have to dampen several different spots on the cloth, repeating the procedure, before you see "nothing" on the cloth. The texture will also stimulate blood flow beneath the surface, so by now, your skin should tingle a little.

Step Three: Apply your nightly skin cream or a skin treatment of choice.

Use the identical cleansing and massaging routine after you get up. After cleansing and massaging, apply a light or rich day cream according to your particular skin needs. The skin will be ready to absorb all the nutrients through the deeply cleansed pores, allowing them to penetrate deeper.

Always apply a moisturizer before you put on your makeup. Even if you don't use makeup, the skin needs a moisturizer anyway. It also helps prevent dirt, bacteria and germs from getting into the pores so easily.

Note: If you want to see how much (and fast) the moisture leaves your skin while you are sleeping at night, try this test: Carefully dampen a tissue and spread it out over your vanity before retiring. The next morning you will find it bone dry. The same thing can happen to the skin of your face and neck.

How to Shrink and Hide Large Pores

There are medical treatments that can help make your pores smaller, if you wish, but you can also camouflage them. The secret is as close by as your makeup tray! We've all heard of applying cold water or a cold compress to shrink pores, but this lasts only until your skin returns to normal temperature after a few minutes. This a classic model's trick and you won't believe how well it works until you try it!

- With a soft makeup sponge apply a foundation on your skin, making sure it fills the pores evenly. Applying in both directions should take care of it. Do not use your fingers, as the makeup will streak and not go on evenly. Also, the heat from your fingers will cause the pores to open up, which you don't want for this procedure: You don't want the makeup to go deeper than needed.

- Take a tissue and lightly remove any excess makeup base on the surface of the skin, leaving the makeup lightly on the skin and in the pores.

- Complete your makeup routine as usual. If you wear cream rouge, this is the time to add it. Then take a clean powder puff with plenty of powder on it and press the powder into the skin and pores over the makeup base. Do not rub the powder around on the skin. When you have done that, gently brush the excess powder off with the powder puff or a large makeup brush. Your skin will look much smoother now.

- Cleanse skin well that night and the next morning.

- Apply an alpha hydroxy acid (AHA) of at least 10% strength—15% is better. AHA helps shrink the pores by regenerating cells under the skin. In the process they expand, thereby causing the skin to become tighter. It also gently sloughs off the top layers making the skin appear smoother. Here's the routine:

  First cleanse with a toner/astringent for deep removal of all oils and bacteria that may remain on the skin and in the pores. It is best to apply this product with a thin, textured washcloth and to use a firm, upward and outward motion. Use a white washcloth to verify that the skin is completely clean.

- At night: Apply AHA to help tighten the pores. Leave on overnight.

- In the morning: Apply a moisturizer cream and makeup as you wish.

Note: *For a permanent reduction of large pores, consult a dermatologist who is affiliated with a hospital. (You can call your local hospital and ask for a recommendation.) Also see Chapter 14: The No-Mistake Makeup School for tricks to hide large pores.*

GETTING RID OF BAD HABITS

Did you know that your behavior patterns are often the main culprits for putting those aging lines in your face? Many people pull down their own facial muscles, for example, through bad habits that they have unconsciously developed over the years. The good news is that by becoming aware of them, you can change them—almost overnight. All it takes is a conscious effort for a few days, then the new habit takes over and it becomes automatic! Have a good friend, your partner, mother, or even your children keep an eye on you for about a week and let you know if you do some of these things.

LARGE PILLOWS

During the night, if your face presses down deep in a large pillow, it will "etch" lines and wrinkles into your skin that will be there when you wake up. It can take several hours before they finally fade away. After a few years these "morning lines" become permanent! So, keep your large pillows for decoration and sleep on a medium-soft, smaller pillow. A baby pillow is even better. The small size allows your face to "control" the pillow and helps prevent the appearance of "pressing" wrinkles around the outer parts of the eyes and mouth.

Sleeping with a large pillow also aids in the development of a double chin by tilting the top of the head forward, thereby pushing your chin down into your chest. But when you sleep on a small pillow, your head remains more in line with your spine, thus allowing your neck and chin to stretch out.

Finally, a large pillow can pull your face muscles down while you sleep. As the bulk of the pillow presses downward on your cheekbone night after night, the muscles below the cheek are pushed down, too. But if you use a small pillow, placing most of it under the chin bone, thereby pushing the cheek muscles up, you'll be giving your face a "lift" every night while you sleep!

Don't worry about having the pillow in place all night long. Whatever happens, it's better than using a large, oversized pillow all night.

FACIAL TICS

Everybody has at least one nervous facial habit or tic! Eventually it leaves its permanent signature on your face. Here are some you would be wise to eliminate.

- Contorting the facial muscles while reading or listening to someone speak.

- Turning the corners of your mouth down while reading. A lot of people do this! Make sure to have someone check you while you're deep into a good book to see if you're one of them! In time, this will become permanent, giving you a sour expression!

- Puckering your lips or "working" your mouth around while you think or work, which will eventually lead to the development of lines around the mouth and chin.

- Frowning, another bad reading habit, can lead to a permanent frown line. Many people also frown when they work intently at their computer. Maybe you need glasses. See an optometrist and find out. Otherwise, learn to relax—taking deep breaths for a while will help you to get rid of this one!

- Rubbing the eyes excessively. I know a person who has this nervous habit. Over the years, the skin around her eyes—both on top and bottom—has become loose and saggy. If your eyes itch frequently, see a doctor. You could be allergic to something. Keep your hands away from your eyes!

BLOWING YOUR NOSE TOO HARD

Be especially careful of this one! If you have a cold, hay fever or sinus problem and your nose is running, it's very easy to rub or twist the skin around your nose and mouth too much. Excessive stretching of the skin can loosen the delicate fibers of the epidermis, causing premature wrinkling! Also, the skin around the base of the nose is very delicate and easily irritated. Too much pressing, twisting and rubbing can cause the tiny blood vessels to rupture, resulting in tiny red lines around the base of your nose. And these are permanent! So use a tissue, but gently!

LEANING YOUR FACE ON YOUR HANDS

Many people lean on their hand with an elbow on the table while talking or listening. Like sleeping on a large pillow, this habit can also lead to the creation of facial lines. But there is no need to hold your head up with your hands! Instead, support your head by keeping your back straight, with your head, neck and spine in alignment. Your neck will look longer, your chin will appear firmer and stronger, and your face will thank you for it in time. Besides, good posture is a must for a great overall appearance.

SPECIAL CARE AROUND THE EYES

The skin under and around your eyes is very delicate and thin, which makes it more sensitive to aging prematurely.

We wake up one morning and all of a sudden we see a tiny line or two around our eyes. Our immediate reaction is, "It just popped up overnight." Wrong! When you see your first line, you should know that it started developing long ago. This is often true of dark circles under the eyes and puffiness, too—they start gradually until, all of a sudden, we notice them.

Proper skin treatment can help prevent these problems from happening, certainly postpone them for many years, and soften the seriousness when they do occur.

Of course, as we grow older, there will be some lines and maybe some puffiness, but they can be greatly reduced. You can still have beautiful skin around your eyes at any age if you make sure to condition and treat it with creams and moisturizers and follow certain guidelines.

■ **Wear sunglasses.** I can't emphasize enough how important it is to protect the delicate skin around your eyes from the sun, not only because the sun dries and wrinkles the skin and hardens the collagen beneath it, but also because it stimulates the production of the pigment melanin, which darkens the skin and exacerbates those dark circles. So it is very, very important to wear good sunglasses. In fact, it's a good idea to carry sunglasses with you all the time, winter or summer. I often wear them even when it's cloudy. Keep an extra pair around. Sunglasses also do another very important thing: They help lessen squinting. Squint lines, also known as crow's-feet, result from exposure to glare and too-bright sunlight. In time, they deepen and eventually become a permanent part of your face! So wearing sunglasses is a must. When purchasing sunglasses, select a brown or gray tint as studies have shown that these neutral colors are best for the health of your eyes, helping to prevent cataracts and macular degeneration.

- **Massage under your eyes.** It's important that the tiny capillaries under the eyes be stimulated. Massaging helps reduce lines, wrinkles, dark circles and puffiness. Take a finger and press firmly, but gently, on one spot in the areas under your eyes. Without lifting your finger make a small rotating motion several times. You can also just press and lift your finger up several times in one spot. Then go to the spot next to it until you have completely massaged the areas under the eye.

- **Sleep the right way.** Puffiness can be caused by an accumulation of fluid, possibly from allergies or sinus problems. Try sleeping with your head slightly elevated so this fluid cannot accumulate as easily. Try this for 2 weeks and monitor the results. I don't believe in sleeping on high pillows in general, as they are not the best for your body alignment. If you decide you need to stay with the higher pillow, make sure your neck is properly supported.

- **Get enough sleep and rest.** Yes, you have heard this before, but it really is true. Try to get 7 or 8 hours of rest each night. Then make up your own mind as to whether this is good for you. Sound sleep provides the best opportunity for your body to repair itself.

- **Deal with allergies.** Many people with allergies frequently rub their eyes, stretching the collagen, fibers and skin in the vicinity. Keep this up and you'll develop loose, maybe even baggy skin around the eyes. See your doctor to get the proper eye drops and treatment, if necessary.

- **Deal with dark circles.** Dark circles can be caused by a number of things, including imbalanced diet and not enough sleep. Work on correcting these. In the meantime, to hide dark circles you can apply a product that covers the dark circles well, yet is light in texture. It contains an ingredient called mica, which causes light reflection that diffuses the dark circles.

- **Reduce stress.** There are some studies that suggest that dark circles are encouraged by stress, which triggers an increase in melanin production under the eyes. If you can't get rid of the stress at the moment, make sure that you are taking enough vitamins, minerals and trace minerals, especially all of the vitamin B family. This can help you deal with the stress better.

- **Check for anemia.** If you are tired for much of the day, have your doctor check you for anemia. This deficiency of red blood cells can cause some discoloration under the eyes.

- **Quit smoking.** Smoking cigarettes slows the blood flow in the face and under the eyes. This means the skin is not getting the proper nourishment it needs to be at its best. Also, every time you draw on a cigarette, you purse your lips. Do this over and over for a long period, and what do you have?—the vertical lines on the skin around your lips that you hate so much.

PREVENT AGING OF NECK AND JOWL LINES

I am often asked if there is anything one can do to keep a young-looking neck and if jowls can be prevented as we grow older. The answer to both questions is yes.

We have all seen women who have youthful skin on their faces, yet their necks look crinkly, rough and course, betraying their age. Here's how to prevent that from happening.

- **Treat the skin of your neck the same way you treat your face, every time.** When you are moisturizing, using a night cream or having a facial treatment, always—and I mean always—include your neck, too.

- **Use sunblock.** The neck has thin skin and the sun will do damage to it quickly, especially if you wear a short hairstyle and the back and sides of your neck are exposed. Be sure to use a sunblock on your neck when outdoors for any length of time. If you are wearing a hat for protection against the sun, it must cover the back and sides of your neck, too. A plain sun visor or cap is not sufficient; you need a brim all the way around. My hair is long, and when I go horseback riding or fly-fishing, I tie it back, so I make sure that my hats are wide enough to protect my neck, too.

- **Give your neck special attention at night when cleansing your face.** Massage it with a light touch and a slow upward motion toward the chin. Use a moisturizer while doing this so your fingers do not "pull or stretch" the skin. This stimulates the small capillaries, bringing more blood and nutrients to the surface for healthier skin.

- **Sleep on a baby pillow.** I have already mentioned the importance of using a pillow the size used on airplanes to prevent morning lines. I also believe the small pillow helps prevent a double chin by keeping the head flatter, in line with the spine, allowing the neck and chin to stretch.

- **Focus on having good posture.** Keep your back straight and chin up. A curved back, chin down will give almost anyone an older-looking neck, and it can produce a double chin, even if you don't actually have one!

- **Adjust your computer screen to the proper height.** A screen that is too low can result in poor posture and a fallen chin—as well as backaches, misalignment of the entire body, and "scrunched up" organs. While sitting with your back straight, head up and chin in, your eyes should be level with the center of the screen. I had a platform built for my desk to raise my computer screen 5 inches so that my eyes look straight into it. I have also moved my computer keyboard higher, so I don't have to look down at it so much, because I'm not a touch typist and have to look at the keys.

Premature jowls are often the result of an overweight body. They develop prematurely because the weight on the face affects the facial muscles, which eventually causes the muscles to "give in" and begin to sag. If you have put on weight and don't like that your jowls or neck are getting too "fleshy," there is really only one surefire remedy—lose weight and you will lose some of the jowl, although my special facial exercises in this chapter can help, too.

When people gain too much weight, no matter how young they are, it usually shows first under the chin and in the stomach. The good news is that when you lose weight, you will lose it in those two places first.

THE IMPORTANCE OF BONE DENSITY

We think of bone loss mostly as affecting the strength and health of the bones in our legs, arms and spine, rendering them brittle or developing osteoporosis. We may worry about losing inches in height. But I'll bet you haven't thought of how it might cause your face to age faster.

If your bone density is not what it should be, as you grow older your skull gets smaller and becomes more brittle, affecting the shape of your face. As you add more weight to a shrinking facial frame, the skin will sag and you will develop deeper lines and wrinkles.

I'm telling you this so you will check with your doctor throughout the years to make sure you are getting enough calcium and/or hormones to keep your bones strong for life…it's not only for your health in general, but for your beauty, too.

Cosmeceutical Products

Alpha Hydroxy Acid (AHA)

Available over the counter, alpha hydroxy acids (AHA) not only rejuvenate the surface of facial skin, but also cause old, flat cells under the skin to regenerate—to become fuller and more youthful. That's because their tiny molecules are small enough to penetrate the skin. They help in rebuilding structural support, causing the skin to "plump up" and appear more youthful. AHA helps restore balance to all types of skin, whether dry or oily, repairs damage from the sun, and helps get rid of that dull, flat look. AHA is known to improve the skin's elasticity while softening and evening out splotches, and diminishing lines and wrinkles. It tightens pores and assists in giving an overall youthful appearance.

I have used AHA products for many years. The most effective ones contain 15% alpha hydroxy acids, which is in the high range of over-the-counter products. The product may contain a combination of several acids, such as glycolic, lactic, citric, tartaric and malic, or it may contain only a single acid.

Tretinoin Cream

Tretinoin (Retin-A) is a prescription cream that helps improve the appearance and texture of the skin. Especially effective for small wrinkles, sun damage and acne, it produces a mild peel on both the superficial (epidermis) and the deep (dermis) skin. It diminishes the effects of sunlight-caused aging by increasing the speed with which the surface cells are replaced. It can also reduce wrinkles, smooth rough patches, and treat areas of darkened skin. Improvements in the skin are visible within 3 to 4 weeks. Brown spots begin to fade after 6 to 8 weeks.

AFTERTHOUGHTS

When I watch my husband shaving his face in the morning, sometimes I think, "thank goodness I don't have to do that." Instead of shaving cream and razor blades, my vanity is fully stocked with wonderful creams and lotions. Every morning, I joyfully use my cleanser and toner/astringent, and I'm so happy that I see a face with smooth, delicate skin staring back at me in the mirror. What does Richard see in his mirror? Stubble! Out comes the razor—poor guy. We women are so lucky. But Richard takes care of his skin, too. He uses an rich aftershave emollient—thick, fragrant, with aloe vera, not one of those alcohol-based lotions—and when he's through, his skin is almost as smooth as mine. Too bad it doesn't last very long before his beard grows out again. So, ladies, no matter what shape your skin is in, count your blessings, and then take my advice and get busy making it better!

CHAPTER 3

YOUTHFUL HANDS, NAILS AND FEET

The most abused parts of your body need your tender loving care.

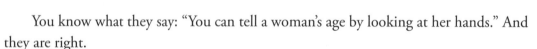

You know what they say: "You can tell a woman's age by looking at her hands." And they are right.

The skin on the back of your hands is extremely thin and delicate. There is almost no fat under it at all, which is why the veins eventually become so visible. As you grow older, any fat that is there will diminish; the skin will become dry and loose, exposing your veins even more. As if that were not enough, you might develop age or sun spots on them as well.

So anyone who wants to project a youthful appearance needs to protect their hands from the sun and from other potentially harmful day-to-day activities like dishwashing, housecleaning, household repairs, etc.

Although my hands look okay for my age, the skin shows signs that I was not as careful as I should have been. I have no arthritis and very flexible fingers, so the shape of both hands is fine, but I did not protect the backs of my hands while I was fly-fishing, riding and gardening. For years I never used gloves or sunblock on them.

As a result, the sun caused some damage to the thin, fair skin, and later on I developed some of those dreaded sun spots. I have used skin lighteners and peeling products to correct the damage with some success.

There was a lot I did not do "back then" that I have since learned and will share with you now. Note to my young friends: Don't ignore this chapter because you have great-looking hands now. Hands start aging when you're not looking. The process starts early and sneaks up on you. If you have darker skin than mine, and think you don't have to worry about the sun on your hands, don't be fooled either. It might not happen to you as quickly, but it will happen.

PRECAUTIONARY MEASURES

GLOVES

Those Victorian ladies who wore gloves whenever they went outside knew something about how to keep their hands smooth and soft. While they may have had different motives—they wanted perfect skin in contrast to the calloused hands of working class women—their method works!

I know because for years now, whenever I go fly-fishing, I pack my fishing gloves with all the other gear. Since I have long fingernails, I wear special gloves for other activities, such as gardening. For horseback riding, I buy inexpensive cotton gloves and cut the fingers off halfway. For the monthly round of golf that I play with my husband, I use specially designed golf gloves that have an opening at the end of each finger so that my nails protrude through them, and I wear them on both hands, even though golfers usually wear only one.

SUNBLOCK

If you have an aversion to wearing gloves while you're doing sports or other outdoor activities, apply a good sunblock to the back of your hands. A sunblock with titanium dioxide and zinc oxide as active ingredients usually produces a white film on the skin, so it doesn't look very pretty, but it provides better protection than those varieties with SPF numbers that protect by absorption of chemicals. Even so, watch it carefully and reapply often. Wearing gloves is best!

Make it a point of noticing for a few weeks how often your hands are exposed to the sun. More than you think, I'll bet! I even keep sunblock in my car, because the hands are often in the sun when driving.

WATER

Another major culprit is water. It will dry out the thin skin of your hands quickly by removing its natural oils, especially when it is warm or hot and soapy, like when you're doing the dishes, bathing babies or washing your hair. Your hands are in contact with water much more than you realize throughout every day.

The best remedy—and we all hate doing it, I know: Wear rubber gloves whenever you can. In addition, keep a hand cream, face cream or body cream—any kind of moisturizing cream—in as many places around your house as you can so you don't have to go looking for one. Keeping the thin skin of your hands constantly moisturized is very important.

BEAUTIFUL, STRONG, HEALTHY NAILS

So many people write to me that they have a serious problem with their nails, even when they keep their nails short. "What to do?" they ask.

Fingernails and toenails are products of your epidermis and are composed of protein (keratin) and sulfur. Each nail grows outward from a nail root that extends back into a groove of skin. Contrary to common belief, the structure of the nails is not related to the structure of bones, and taking extra calcium or gelatin will not strengthen brittle nails.

One of the most common causes of nail change is fungus, which can cause the nails to crack, peel and change color and texture. These infections are not always easy to treat, and the sooner you deal with them, the better. Seek professional help if symptoms persist.

Fingernails normally grow at the rate of 1/8 inch a month, approximately 2 or 3 times faster than toenails. Growth slows as we age. Sudden or significant changes in the appearance of the nails can be a first sign of illness. If your fingernails begin to change texture or color, you may need to see a doctor.

Abnormal or unhealthy nails may be the result of a local injury, a glandular deficiency such as hypothyroidism, or a lack of certain nutrients. Thus, a protein deficiency can cause opaque white bands to appear on the nails. Insufficient amounts of protein, vitamin A or iron slows down the rate of nail growth and may also result in dryness and brittleness. Lack of B vitamins causes nails to become fragile; horizontal or vertical ridges may appear. Frequent hangnails usually indicate an inadequate intake of vitamin C, folic acid and protein.

White spots can be caused by a zinc or iron deficiency. If they appear, a zinc supplement should be considered. Do not take an iron supplement, however, without consulting your doctor since an overabundance of iron can cause toxicity

> ZINC is found in dairy products, eggs, beans, nuts and pumpkin seeds.
>
> IRON can be obtained by eating red meat, fish, poultry, lentils and beans.

Any nail abnormality can be an indication that the diet is not adequate, so eating well-balanced meals supplying all essential nutrients is very important.

Fingernail Advice

Here are some measures that will help make your nails strong and resilient, and keep them that way.

- Use your fingers, not your nails, to pick things up. This, of course, is easier said than done! If you have long nails, use the sides of your fingers.

- Carry a small Band-Aid in your handbag. If a nail cracks, put it on immediately, then mend your nail as soon as you return home. You can buy a "mending kit" in almost any drugstore.

- Wear rubber gloves whenever you use soap and water or do any kind of manual activity. Make sure they are larger than your usual glove size.

- Always protect your nails with a coat of some type of polish, even clear polish.

- For extra strength and proper conditioning, use a liquid collagen product on the surface of the nail. Also apply a nail hardener until your nails become stronger. Both of these products are available in a nail polish-type bottle.

GIVE YOURSELF A PROFESSIONAL MANICURE AT HOME

Allow yourself about an hour and assemble everything you need before you begin:

> clean hand towel
> cuticle cutter if you need one
> hydrogen peroxide
> cotton
> polish remover
> bowl of soapy water
> emery board
> cuticle oil
> orange sticks—sometimes called cuticle sticks
> nail polish
> top-coat sealer

1. Clean off old polish with cotton pads soaked in polish remover. Take care not to push the old polish into the cuticle. Start from the base of the nail and work toward the tip.

2. Be sure your nails are dry before you file them. Begin at the side with the emery board and sweep to the center; never use a "saw-like" motion. Don't round off the nails too much, for that can cause them to break easily. The longer your nails, the more "square" they should be. But always round off the corners a little so they look more natural.

3. Soak your fingers in warm soapy water for 2 to 3 minutes to help clean the nails and soften the cuticles.

4. Clean your nails with the orange stick dipped in hydrogen peroxide.

5. Apply cuticle remover or oil. Wrap a tiny piece of cotton around the tip of the orange stick and gently work it around each nail to loosen the cuticle. This is also the time to clip away any loose cuticle tissue. Do this gently or you may hurt yourself or cause hangnails.

6. Apply a base coat. This semi-transparent "polish" puts a smooth protective layer on the nail and is especially helpful for brittle and weak nails. Use strong brush strokes from the base of the nail to the tip.

7. After the base coat is dry, apply your polish (of course, it can be clear). Thin it down, if necessary, with polish remover. This is one of the secrets for professional-looking nails.

   Wait until each coat of polish dries a little before applying the next; if it's thin polish, it won't take long. Brush the color across the base of your nail first, keeping clear of the cuticle, then make 2 strokes along the edges from base to tip. Finally, fill in the middle with one strong stroke from the base to the tip. Never go back over wet polish or you will get ridges. If you smudge a nail, apply a little polish remover while the nail is still wet, then smooth it over ever so lightly with the nail polish brush.

8. Apply top-coat sealer. Sealers prolong the wear of your polish, delay chipping and make your nails thicker and stronger. Allow your nails to dry for 20 minutes.

Younger, Prettier Feet at Any Age

Considering how much time we spend on our feet, it is certainly worth taking good care of them. Make sure they're healthy, and yes, even beautiful, especially during the warm summer months when you'll want to slip into sandals or even go barefoot.

There are several things that can be done to help take care of tired, sore and unattractive feet.

- Wear shoes that fit well and feel comfortable. This is especially important for any shoe that you wear for long periods of time, including shoes that you put on for exercise. Pointy shoes and shoes that pinch can lead to other foot problems such as bunions, calluses and hammertoe. You should never have to "break in" shoes. If they are uncomfortable in the store, don't buy them.

- Be careful with high heels. They can be dangerous to your health. It takes some time to show the ill effects, and most people don't make the connection between joint pain in knees and "killer" stilettos. Once they do, it's usually too late—the damage is done.

- Orthopedists have warned women for years that high heels can contribute to the development of corns, calluses, knee pain, sprained and broken ankles, arthritis and the breakdown of cartilage surrounding the knee, not to mention back problems. The reason is that high heels produce an unnatural positioning of the feet and improper distribution of weight. Wear high-heeled shoes sparingly.

Research also shows that the fashionable wide high heels are just as damaging over time.[4] While they are better for your feet, they increase the risk of developing osteoarthritis in the knees just as much as narrow heels do.

Shoes with heels of 1½ to 1¾ inches, a bit squared off so the toes have room, are the safest. Flat shoes without arch supports worn all the time can also be damaging.

- Indulge in a foot soak. It can do wonders. Swelling is often caused by too much fluid being retained in the body. When you soak your feet in Epsom salt, it draws water out along with toxins, reducing swelling, relaxing muscles and helping with exfoliation. It also helps aching feet, removes odors and softens rough skin. Plus, it feels good. Add ½ cup of Epsom salt to a large pan of very warm water. Soak feet for 15 minutes or as long as it feels right. Rinse and dry.

- Next, rub in an oil or body lotion of your choice to moisturize the skin—either will work. Apply again before going to bed.

Caring For Your Feet

If you often have foot odor, bacterial or fungus problems, you may not be washing your feet properly. Don't imagine that soap and water is always enough. A good number of foot issues could be solved with proper washing.

Use a soft scrub brush as well as a loofah. Wash the entire foot with the loofah and a lot of lather, then take the scrub brush to clean the nails really well. Antibacterial soap is available if you have odor or other bacterial issues. If you have a fungal problem, you can also buy fungal soap, but fungal drops that are applied directly on the fungus are best.

If you have a lot of calluses or dry, cracked patches, you can use a pumice stone or a foot file to get rid of them. Make sure the feet are very dry when you do this.

Clip your toenails. The best time is when they are softened by the water. Clip them straight across to make sure that you avoid encouraging ingrown nails.

For pretty feet, follow the directions on page 46 to give yourself a professional pedicure at home.

Apply moisturizer on your feet as well as your toenails and massage it in. Then use a cloth to wipe the moisturizer off the toenails.

Now go out and buy yourself a new pair of sandals that show off your glamorous toes and feet!

AFTERTHOUGHTS

I have never been big on jewelry. I see many women wearing a couple of bracelets, rings and other jewelry on their hands at the same time. It works for them, but that's not me. However, I do love well kept nails and toes. They are more important to me than any number of diamonds on my fingers or fancy toe rings. No amount of jewelry will cover up neglected hands or feet. But, of course, I would never refuse the diamonds!

Chapter 4

TEETH AND GUMS FOR LIFE

Many Americans lose some or all of their teeth by age 45 unnecessarily.

When you were young, chances are your mother constantly reminded you to brush your teeth. She really should have told you to brush your teeth *and massage your gums*.

Most of us start out with strong healthy teeth and gums. The way you take care of them day-to-day determines whether you keep them for life. Yet 43% of Americans have lost some or even all of their teeth by the time they've reached age 45; and that's a shame, because they are really designed to last a lifetime. Neglect or lack of information is almost always the culprit.

When people lose their teeth, they often think it is part of the normal aging process. Let me tell you—it is not. If your parents lost their teeth, it was most likely because of neglect, not old age. It is generally accepted by the medical community that tooth loss can be prevented through education, early diagnosis and regular dental care.

You have control over the health of your gums and teeth. If you still have all or most of your teeth, start to take care of them now and keep them forever.

When I became a model, two of my upper front teeth were off center. A tooth had been taken out at an early age because it had grown in the wrong way, and the resulting gap caused the rest of my teeth to shift to the right. I had those two front teeth capped to correct the imbalance. Later, I had others capped for cosmetic reasons, but I have never had a serious tooth or gum problem in all my 75 years. Recently my dentist told me that I have the healthy gums of someone in their 20s and to keep on doing whatever it is I'm doing. I intend to.

THE IMPORTANCE OF GUM CARE

Sometimes harmful bacteria can build up under your gum line and cause an infection known as periodontal disease or gum disease. All periodontal disease begins with gingivitis—inflammation, swelling and bleeding gum tissue caused by a buildup of dental plaque—which in time can lead to tooth loss if not treated. It is necessary to remove dental plaque daily through proper brushing and cleansing, and by periodic visits to a dental hygienist.

Replacing teeth is very expensive, and I've been told regular false teeth, such as bridges and dentures, don't work as well as your original, natural ones. Replacement tooth implants do function as well; however, basic implants cost $1,250 to $3,000 each, and the procedures can escalate to between $15,000 and $30,000, depending on location, complexity and need for bone or gum restoration work.

Let me say right here that you should never go to bed without brushing and cleaning your teeth each night. If you heard this as a child, pay attention. It is still true, no matter your age.

Actually, it's not the cleaning of the teeth that's so important to prevent gum disease; it's the removal of all traces of food and drink between each tooth and from under the gums, so that bacteria can't develop.

I believe that stimulating the gums in order to speed the blood flow is very important for the health of the area surrounding each tooth—its gums and roots—and helps keep them firm and strong. Using dental floss and/or a dental water jet is also very important because they stimulate the gums, as well as remove food and bacteria….do not go to bed without removing food and bacteria.

One positive note is that gum disease might be reversible if caught in time.

My Personal Routine

I brush my teeth and gums well when I get up in the morning, making sure I include both the inside and outside of the gums around the teeth. At night I do the same thing again, but also use a dental water jet, which finds more particles to remove, even after just brushing.

Personally, I have never flossed. When a new dentist sees my teeth and gums, the first thing he remarks is, "I guess you floss twice a day." I love to reply, "I never floss. I use a Waterpik®!" I'm not against flossing…and I don't own any stock in Waterpik. It just does the job for me. I usually add a little anti-bacterial mouthwash to the water jet, for added assistance and freshness.

I also take vitamin B complex and a good antioxidant vitamin, mineral and trace mineral every day, which are good for the whole body, as well as teeth and gums.

Many people need to use both floss and a water jet—especially when they have waited too long to start caring for their teeth and gums. But whatever it takes, do it! The alternative is likely to be painful and very expensive.

Good Bone Density Helps You Keep Your Teeth

The bone of your jaw anchors your teeth. Loss of calcium leads to loss of the bone surrounding the teeth and their roots, resulting in teeth loosening and even falling out.

Infection is another common reason for bone loss. If it spreads to the nerve in the root and into the surrounding jaw, it will eventually destroy some of the bone. The weaker your bone density, the more bone will be destroyed.

Note: Don't drink too much soda or coffee, and drink alcoholic beverages in moderate amounts, or not at all. They are all associated with weakened bones when consumed in large amounts and on a daily basis. Also avoid extreme dieting, which can rob bones of important nutrients.

To keep your bones strong, see your doctor for more information. Tell him you would like to have a bone density test. You may have to push a little because some doctors don't think to do it on their own unless you're over 65. Depending on the results, you may need to exercise more and consider adjusting your eating habits.

Nutrition for Teeth, Gums and Jaws

Your body stops building bone at about age 30. After that you need a calcium-rich diet to keep them strong.

VITAMIN A and C is found in milk, yogurt, cheese, fresh fruit and vegetables.

VITAMIN D helps the body absorb calcium. Good sources are salmon, mackerel and tuna.

Cosmetic Procedures for Teeth

Tooth enamel discoloration and staining can be caused by coffee, tea and cigarettes. People who drink large amounts of cola soft drinks can experience similar staining.

There are other factors that can affect the color of an individual's teeth. Genetics plays a role. Some people have naturally brighter enamel than others. Disease and certain medications also can cause discoloration. If you suspect that there is an underlying medical cause for your teeth discoloration, be sure to inform your cosmetic dentist.

There are many methods available to obtain whiter teeth, but no matter which you choose, peroxide is the active whitening agent used in all bleaching gels, in various concentrations, from as little as 3% in home remedy products to 15% when done professionally. Your choice depends on how much you are willing to spend, how quickly you want results, how white you want your teeth, and how long you want it to last.

Although some people may experience sensitivity to certain concentrations of bleaching gel, it is generally mild and short lived, so you can feel safe and confident using a teeth whitening gel to give you a bright, dazzling smile. There has been some concern that some processes damage tooth enamel and cause gum disease, but studies have produced no evidence of that.

Results vary, so, if you want whiter teeth, I suggest you consult your dentist. But first, here's some advance knowledge about the processes available so that you can make an informed decision depending on your need and how much money you wish to spend.

Laser-Activated Systems

Dentists or professional practitioners use a whitening system such as BriteSmile or Zoom. These involve 90-minute sessions in which hydrogen peroxide gel is applied to your teeth and activated with ultraviolet light. The process is repeated 3 times at 15-minute intervals. The results are immediate and amazing with up to 9 or 10 shades of lightening.

The procedure comes with a touch-up kit for you to take home. If you follow the directions and use the touch-up kit when a stain appears, and especially if you don't smoke and avoid a lot of caffeine and other stain-producing foods, you can maintain beautifully white teeth indefinitely.

The cost ranges from $400 to $600.

Custom Trays

To create custom whitening trays, your dentist will take an impression of your teeth and have trays made for your uppers and lowers that will fit perfectly over your teeth. He will then provide the whitening material, usually at 9 to 10% concentration of hydrogen peroxide, for you to place in the trays at home and position over your teeth for 30 to 60 minutes once a day until your teeth have whitened to the desired shade. Average time required for optimum results is 20 to 30 days.

The cost ranges from $300 to $500.

Over-the-Counter Whiteners

Caution: One of the big advantages of professional teeth whitening is that you will always receive an examination and a professional cleaning before the procedure. This prevents any possible damage from the peroxide penetrating cavities or other periodontal openings. Therefore, before embarking on any home remedy, I suggest you have an examination and professional cleaning first, or, if you're certain you have no cavities, make sure you give yourself a thorough cleaning and flossing.

All over-the-counter home whitening systems are less effective and take longer for results to appear than professional treatment. However, they are far less expensive and the results can be quite acceptable.

Methods include trays, whitening strips and pens that cost around $35 or less.

Natural Teeth Whitening

Generally, beware of natural home remedies. Some teeth whitening home remedies are downright dangerous to your teeth, while others may be worth your time.

Three common home remedies are detailed below.

- **Baking soda.** The process of brushing teeth with a baking soda and salt mixture has been around for a long time. It can actually be effective in removing stains, especially with the help of peroxide. Although not as effective a whitener as the more highly concentrated gels, it is inexpensive and works as a good maintenance product, especially if you mix in some of your toothpaste to improve the taste.

- **Lemon juice.** Brushing teeth with lemon juice, or rubbing the peel across the teeth, is one of the most frequently mentioned ways to whiten teeth naturally. Unfortunately, it is also one of the worst. The citric acid in the juice robs your tooth enamel of calcium—not good, considering that teeth will decay much faster that way. Lemon juice can also strip away the tooth enamel until it is damaged beyond repair.

- **Strawberries.** Another home remedy using fruit involves mashing strawberries into a paste and brushing your teeth with it. While it might taste good, it is almost as harmful as lemon juice.

Tooth Veneers

Veneers are thin pieces of specially shaped porcelain or plastic that are glued over the front of your teeth. Used for severely discolored, chipped or crooked teeth, or for unwanted or uneven spaces, they require the dentist to remove much less of the tooth than crowns. Veneers also cost less, won't stain, and should last from 10 to 15 years.

Dental Implants

If you're missing a tooth or all of your teeth, talk to your dentist about implants. As long as you have enough bone in the area to facilitate the anchorage of the implants, this procedure can yield great results. If you don't have enough, a bone graft may be necessary. The implant itself will last a lifetime, but its crown will last 10 to 15 years.

Tooth Bonding

Bonding can lighten stains, close up minor gaps, correct crooked teeth and restore decayed teeth. Bonding covers flaws by applying a thin coating of a plastic material on the front surface of your teeth, followed by a high-intensity light which hardens the plastic, after which the surface is finely polished. Bonding lasts about 10 years.

Caps

Caps can be used with teeth that are no longer structurally sound due to lost fillings, decay below a filling, or chipping and cracking of the enamel. If the entire surface of the tooth is a problem, but the root system is intact, a cap might be appropriate. Caps are used also for cosmetic reshaping of teeth.

AFTERTHOUGHTS

Your dentist can tell you how healthy your gums are no matter what your age. The dentists I have seen over the years in New York, Texas and Florida all have told me that they wish they could bottle and sell whatever it is I do.

If your dentist doesn't tell you the state of your gums, you should ask. Unless his answer is "excellent," you should be concerned. If he says, "OK," they aren't. "OK" doesn't cut it with gums if you want to keep your teeth for a lifetime. "OK" means your gums are not as healthy or as strong as they should be. Find out what you need to do to get them to "excellent."

CHAPTER 5

GORGEOUS HAIR ALL YOUR LIFE

Another birthday won't make your hair look older...
lack of information will.

It wasn't always like this. When I was 29 and a model in New York City, I was concerned about the length of my hair. In fact, whenever a client wanted to have my hair shortened because they needed a certain look for an ad, I refused. I figured that when I reached the ripe old age of 30, I'd be required to cut my hair short or risk looking silly as an older woman with long hair. I lost a few bookings because of it, but I wanted to have long hair as long as I could.

Well, as you can see, I changed my mind about long hair on older women. I still keep it long even at age 75. Long hair may not be for everyone, I just happen to like it for me. I learned, and now I preach, we can look and be younger as long as we wish, if we take care of ourselves

A beautiful head of hair speaks to a woman's good health, glamour and allure. It's also a symbol of distinction and a window into her personality. A woman's hair can be of short, long or medium length; red, black, blond, brown or gray in color; elegantly or simply styled. But it must be healthy and good-looking.

A change of style or color can satisfy a whim or a desire to show off a new look, revealing a "new you," as it were. Strong, healthy, dazzling hair gives a woman a sense of well-being. As an important feature of her femininity and beauty, it can also be a source of peace of mind and greater self confidence.

When I was on a commercial shoot as a model, there was no excuse for dull or unhealthy-looking hair. Not only would bad hair get you thrown off the set, but word would spread throughout the industry, and you would find it more difficult to get bookings, and certainly none for hair ads. When a model is paid big bucks, she is expected to look perfect for the shoot, no matter what, and her hair is a very important aspect of her appearance.

Many people believe that the older they get, the older their hair should look. But that is baloney! Beautiful, healthy, strong, dazzling hair has nothing to do with age! Everyone is capable of having glamorous and youthful-looking hair.

A Profile of Your Hair

The 100,000 or so hairs on your head are composed of nitrogen, sulfur, water, amino acids and iron traces. Women's hair lasts about 25% longer than men's before it falls out to be replaced, a process that takes 2 to 6 years. Hair grows faster in summer and, strangely, faster at night.

Each hair is rooted in a follicle, a singular depression in your scalp. In a healthy scalp, when that hair falls out, there is already a new hair shaft ready to replace it.

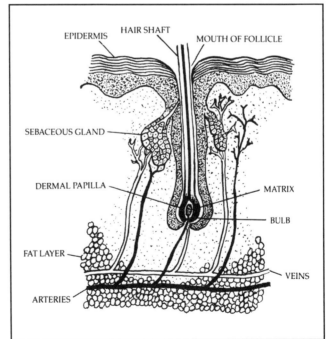

New hair growth starts in the papilla. It grows under an existing hair shaft and eventually pushes it out. Meanwhile, tiny blood vessels feed both follicle and papilla with nutrients and oxygen, and carry away waste and carbon dioxide.

Massaging the scalp helps keep the blood flowing to the papilla. Without blood the papilla will die. But if you stimulate and nourish the scalp properly, you can invigorate the papilla and produce strong, healthy hair again. Proper vitamins and minerals will help in the production of a richer flow of blood, so the food you feed your body can make a big difference to your hair.

Each follicle also has its own gland to manufacture the vital oils needed for healthy hair. This gland secretes enough oil to fill in the "cracks" in the outer layer of each hair (the cuticle). These surface fissures are what make the hair look dull and dry. By filling them in, the exterior becomes smooth again. This, in turn, allows it to reflect light more evenly and gives it that special shine we all associate with healthy, beautiful hair.

Massage Your Scalp for Thickness and Strength

Scalp massage is very important for healthy hair that's strong and growing, and for oily hair, which tends to have more sluggish scalp circulation than other types of hair. The older we get, the more our circulation slows, making scalp massage even more essential.

The goal is to bring a greater flow of blood to your hair follicles and papillae and to make your scalp more flexible. Massage will also speed the removal of oil and dead cells that form debris on the surface, hardening and sticking to the scalp, reducing circulation and eventually destroying hair roots. Often, this debris can't be seen by the naked eye because it can form in the skin's pores.

1. **Move the scalp.** Once or twice a day, take both hands and place your fingertips on your scalp without bending them. Do not push the hair, but keep the fingers firmly on one spot, pushing the whole scalp in a circular motion for a few seconds. You will feel a large section of your scalp moving around. That's good! Now place your fingers in a new area and repeat the motion until you have covered the entire scalp and your head tingles and feels warm (from increased circulation). Pay special attention to any thinning areas or bald spots—these areas need even more stimulation.

2. **Scratch the scalp.** Now, using your fingertips or fingernails, or a large wide-toothed comb, create a vigorous rubbing motion. This time you are not "moving your scalp" but rather "scratching" it until your head tingles and feels warm. Pay special attention to the top of your head and

your temples, which are the most difficult areas for attaining good blood circulation.

3. **Pull the hair.** Next, take a clump of hair in each hand and pull on it gently but firmly for 3 counts. Release and repeat until you have done all the hair on your scalp.

When you start this treatment, in the first week or 2 you'll see some hair loss, but don't worry—those hairs were coming out anyway. New, healthier hair will replace it. You can be sure that with this massage you are taking charge and changing the condition of the hair follicles, strengthening them, making them healthier. This allows new hair growth in the formerly unhealthy follicles. If the follicles have been deprived for several years, new growth cannot develop.

Before starting this program, part your hair in the middle and hold both sides down flat and tight. Look closely and see how many tiny new hairs are coming in. If you're having hair problems, it may be only a few. After 2 or 3 weeks, repeat this process. You should see many more new hairs. They will appear short and "singed" on the ends; they represent the beginning of new, stronger growth. At the same time, your roots have become more nourished so that the old hair is stronger and healthier, too.

I have seen the success of this treatment so many times…but you must stay with it until your hair is as thick and strong as you like it.

Nutrition for Hair

Hair is a mirror of your general health. As the years go by it's almost impossible to eat enough foods rich in vitamins and minerals for the kind of strength, thickness, shine, vitality and growth your hair had when you were younger. You can have beautiful, healthy hair at any age if you compensate for what it is lacking by eating well-balanced meals and taking nutritional supplements.

VITAMIN A can be found in dark green vegetables like spinach and broccoli.

OMEGA-3 FATTY ACIDS can be found in salmon.

WHY HAIR TURNS GRAY

When your first gray hairs start to appear, it can shake you up. But gray hair is flattering if it is a "white-gray," shiny and well cared for. But of course, that's my opinion. I have seen beautiful salt-and-pepper color hair too…the key is keeping it shiny and healthy-looking.

The color of your hair is determined by the amount of the pigments eumelanin and pheomelanin in your follicles (they are 2 types of melanin—the same pigment that's in your skin). The more eumelanin you have, the darker your hair will be; the more pheomelanin, the redder. As you grow older, the pigment cells gradually die. As the melanin decreases, your hair becomes more transparent and turns gray, silver or white.

If you like your original hair color, there are lotions and color foams that will cover the gray without changing your own natural hair color. They will fade away after about 4 to 6 washings, but as you continue to use them, they will hold up better.

If you decide to go with gray, you will definitely want to avoid yellow discoloration. The best way to do that is to use what is called a "gray enhancer." If your hair has a lot of yellow discoloration, apply platinum tones to help tone it down. If you want to deepen its shade and even it out, look into smoky tones. These gray enhancers wash out so you can easily change to a lighter or darker shade when you reapply them.

DEALING WITH DIFFERENT KINDS OF HAIR

Regardless of the kind of hair you have, you should always do the following.

- Wash your hair frequently. Try a lemon or vinegar rinse. This will reduce the amount of excess oil.

- After washing, blot hair dry with a towel. If you use a dryer, put it on a cooler setting. Heat can stimulate production in your oil glands.

- Choose a hairstyle that is worn off the face.

DRY HAIR

- When washing your hair, use a shampoo made especially for dry hair.

- Apply conditioner, making sure to use one that will penetrate the hair, rather than merely coating it. Read the label: Look for a conditioner that contains botanicals such as avocado, jojoba oil, shea butter, panthenol, silicone or dimethicone.

- After washing, blot the hair dry with a towel, but do not rub it too vigorously, since you might cause breakage. If you use a dryer, put it on a cooler setting. Although heat can increase oil production in the scalp, it's not likely in a dry head of hair, and it can dry out any oil that might be there and render your hair more vulnerable to breakage.

- Avoid harsh chemical processes, such as coloring or straightening, and very hot rollers.

- If you use rollers, use end papers (these can be folded tissue). Avoid sponge-type rollers which will absorb oil from the hair.

- If you have a dry scalp, once a week, apply a light oil or cream to your scalp for treatment.

- After a wash, use a comb with large gaps between rounded teeth. Part the hair and work in sections, blotting it dry. Remember to work from the end of your hair inward to the scalp. You can press your fingertips firmly on the roots while you work at untangling the ends.

BABY-FINE HAIR

This type of hair can be a challenge. It is hard to manage because it is limp, light and fly-away. It doesn't hold a curl very well, splits and breaks easily, and is full of static electricity. Baby-fine hair quickly becomes dull and oily after shampooing and has a tendency to separate because it collects moisture, oil and dirt so quickly.

Here are some simple rules to help you handle such hair.

- Get a good, blunt cut. Baby-fine hair just doesn't do well in layers. All one length is easiest to handle. If you want to wear it long, by all means do so, but make sure it's long enough to wear pulled back for those days when it's just impossible to handle. Also, remember to get regular trims every 4 to 6 weeks.

- Wash your hair as often as you like, but use a hair body builder, hair thickener or setting lotion for added body and weight. For the "firmest" set, dry your hair well with a towel and then apply the setting lotion to hair and set. Try a light conditioner if hair is too fly-away.

- If you like, color or tint your hair (streaking and frosting helps, too). Color-treated hair has more body and is easier to handle. But because fine hair needs the gentlest touch, stick with the more "natural" coloring agents.

- A soft body wave will add fullness and make your hair much easier to handle. But if you color your hair, the body wave may cause breakage. Check with a reliable hairdresser.

- Eat a diet high in protein or take protein supplements.

THICK HAIR

The good news about thick hair is that it is probably strong enough to withstand harsh chemical processes such as straightening.

- If you set your hair, use large rollers for a large and loose curl (small curls will make your hair look even thicker).

- Combing and brushing will take a little longer, but a little patience will pay off with a beautiful head of well-groomed hair. Comb through all tangles, using your fingers to help separate them.

AFRICAN-AMERICAN HAIR

Most hair of African-American women is quite dry, surprisingly delicate and more susceptible to harsh treatment, so my advice regarding dry hair applies here, too. In addition, here are a few special pointers from some of the beautiful black models I've worked with. They'll make it possible for you to get the most out of your hair, while keeping it strong and healthy.

- For dried-out hair that's been abused by chemical straighteners, try this completely natural treatment: Mix equal parts sesame oil, castor oil and light mineral oil. Add 3 teaspoons liquid lecithin. Section hair and apply the mixture to your scalp with a cotton pad. Pour any remaining oil over hair and massage it well into scalp. Cover your head tightly with plastic. Let sit for 15 to 20 minutes and shampoo out, making sure to rinse thoroughly. The oils will give your hair a lovely sheen, while the lecithin will help the hair repair itself.

- Trim hair regularly to maintain the shape.

- Be sure to massage your scalp frequently to increase blood flow.

- For maximum fullness, use a pick to separate and fluff hair up.

- Many black women look lovely in hair a few shades lighter than their own natural color—for example, light browns or auburns—which can enhance their particular skin tones. But because black hair is so porous, be very careful when applying color yourself. Follow directions to the letter, and don't forget to perform a "strand test" before doing the entire head.

SPECIAL PROBLEMS

SPLIT ENDS

This is the bad news: The only cure for split ends is to trim them off. The longer you leave a split alone, the farther it will travel up the hair shaft. The good news is that you can prevent split ends from occurring again.

- Use a shampoo formulated specifically for dry hair.

- Apply a protein conditioner after every shampoo. If your hair is oily, use it only on the ends of hair. Once a month, deep condition.

- Always use end papers when setting hair (folded tissues are fine).

- Don't use a hot hair dryer, hot rollers or hot combs more than once a week. If you can, use a medium temperature.

- Comb out wet hair with a wide-toothed comb and start at the ends, working your way gently to the scalp.

SUNBURNED HAIR

Sun-damaged hair is dry, stiff and dull. It's difficult to control, and it sometimes breaks. Another symptom is faded-looking color that often varies from area to area.

- Use a protein conditioner after shampooing.

- Cover your hair with a scarf or hat when out in the hot sun for a long time.

- Brush and comb sun-damaged hair gently—especially when wet.

- Avoid the use of hot combs, hot rollers and hand dryers. Your hair has had enough "heat" for awhile.

- For severely damaged hair, try this easy home treatment: Heat 1/2 cup of olive oil in a saucepan until just warm (not hot). Apply to your head, making sure that the entire shaft of the hair is covered from root to tip. Wrap your hair tightly in a thin towel or piece of plastic for 10 minutes. If this doesn't work, set the hair dryer on "warm" and use for 10 minutes. Then, wash with shampoo, rinsing several times to make sure that you've removed all the oil.

DANDRUFF

Dandruff may not be fatal, but it sure is embarrassing, as all those TV commercials remind us. It is probably the most common condition afflicting the hair and scalp, and it occurs with all types of hair—normal, oily or dry. While it is perfectly natural for excess cells of the scalp to die and flake off, in much the same way as individual hairs die and fall out, when this shedding process becomes excessive, then it becomes a problem.

Except in the most severe cases, for which the medical term is seborrhea, dandruff is generally attributed to a faulty diet, emotional tension, hormonal imbalance or the improper use of haircare products.

There are a variety of treatments, depending on whether your hair is oily, dry or normal.

DANDRUFF AND OILY HAIR

Diet plays an important part in controlling dandruff in oily hair. Too much chocolate, nuts, shellfish, iodized salt, butter and fried foods have been related to an increase in dandruff. Alcohol, too, can aggravate the condition. So, my first suggestion is that you eliminate these foods from your diet completely for a one-month test, or at least keep them down to a minimum. If you don't see any improvement, try the following regimen.

- Massage your scalp at least once a day, preferably in the morning. Finish by brushing your hair with long, smooth strokes. This will remove much of the loose dandruff that might fall off during the day and settle on your shoulders and clothes. Be sure to keep your brush and comb very clean! Don't allow any dandruff to remain in them.

- To remove the accumulated dead cells and oil, use a strong sulfur dandruff shampoo. Then switch back to your regular shampoo. Too much sulfur can make the condition worse. While you are using the sulfur shampoo, wash your hair more often and replace fried and fatty foods with fresh fruits and vegetables. Follow instructions on the label on how long you should use the product.

- Before each shampoo, moisten a piece of sterile gauze with witch hazel. Then, part and section your hair and rub it with the gauze. Try to cover as much of the scalp as possible. After that, wash your hair as usual, making sure to rinse thoroughly so that none of the witch hazel remains.

Note: Make sure not to wet the gauze too much and squeeze it out before applying to the scalp. Witch hazel can be harmful to your eyes and facial skin (if it is dry) if it should drip.

DANDRUFF AND DRY HAIR

Again, my first advice is to check your diet. You may need to eat more foods like pork, shellfish, nuts and butter. If you're trying to lose weight, this new regimen doesn't have to sabotage your diet. For example, 2 or 3 pats of butter a day or 2 strips of bacon should be enough to correct your dryness problem while adding only about 100 calories to your daily intake. Shellfish is particularly good because it contains enough oils to equalize the balance of your body, and it is low in calories. You could also take an omega-3 fatty acid supplement.

To help your immediate problem, you should follow these steps.

- Massage your scalp once a day to loosen the dandruff scales and then brush thoroughly with long, smooth strokes to remove them.

- Shampoo daily with products recommended especially for dry hair. Do not use an anti-dandruff shampoo or any product containing sulfur.

- Before each shampoo, heat some olive oil in a small saucepan until it is warm, but not hot. Section your hair carefully with a comb and apply the warm olive oil with a clean gauze pad to each part. When you have pretty well covered the entire head, massage the remainder of the oil into the scalp. Now, wrap your hair carefully in a light towel—if possible, warm it with a hair dryer—and keep it on for 15 minutes. Then shampoo your hair as usual and finish off with a warm water rinse to make sure that all oil is removed.

DANDRUFF AND NORMAL HAIR

Severe dandruff in normal hair is an indication that all is not well—and the problem may go deeper than your scalp. When itching accompanies dandruff, do not scratch. Instead, rub the scalp gently with your fingertips. Do not use your nails!. Scratching this sensitive area can result in an irritated scalp, which can eventually become red and thicken, restricting the natural flow of oil from the pores. When untreated, this condition can spread to the face and neck, at which point you had better see a dermatologist. Frequent scratching of the scalp can lead to infection, which may destroy the hair follicles to the point where you will end up with a permanent bald spot.

Dandruff in normal hair is usually the result of emotional tension, hormonal imbalance and/or a diet too rich in sweets, starches, oil, junk food and soft drinks, resulting in a deficiency in vitamin B. To treat dandruff due to a poor diet, it is very important that you take a natural vitamin and mineral supplement. Also, try the following routine.

- Massage your scalp once a day. Then brush your hair thoroughly with long, smooth strokes to remove the loosened flakes.

- Shampoo daily with shampoo for normal hair.

- Once a week, take 1 or 2 egg yolks (depending on how much hair you have) and mix them with a small amount of water. Beat well. Gently rub this liquid into a dry scalp after the hair has been carefully brushed. Massage gently and then let sit for 20 to 30 minutes. Rinse thoroughly for one of the best "egg shampoos" you'll ever get.

Hair Loss and Remedies

Just as our skin loses elasticity and becomes thinner as we age, so does our scalp. As a result of diminished flexibility and tightening passageways, the little blood vessels just below the skin's surface can no longer provide a full, rich, fast-flowing blood stream to the follicles, thus depriving them of essential nutrients and oxygen. Let this continue and it's a death sentence for the thick, shiny, healthy hair of your youth.

Another reason for thinning hair may be a hormonal imbalance. Testosterone, the male hormone that is also present in women, produces a by-product called dihydrotestosterone (DHT) that causes hair loss. But the female hormones, estrogen and progesterone, both block the effect of DHT on hair—unless there's a deficiency in them, which can happen after pregnancy and during menopause. The answer to this could be hormone replacement therapy (HRT) under the proper guidance of a competent doctor.

Sometimes the appearance of bald spots or thinning hair has nothing to do with your diet or the condition of your hair. Rather, they can be the result of undue pressure on the scalp, or mistreating your hair in ways you might not realize. For example:

- Sleeping with rollers tightly anchored with pins or cups over and over may lead to balding wherever the pressure points are (brush rollers are especially dangerous). In the process, you are cutting off the vital supply lines that bring food and oxygen to the hair roots. As a result, your hair will start to grow more and more slowly, and eventually fall out.

- Tight ponytails worn day in and day out also put too much pressure on the scalp, reducing vital circulation. Hair loss eventually occurs around the hairline. Changing your hairstyle to a loose one and massaging the area daily will usually stop this kind of balding.

- Dandruff can cause hair loss if it is too severe. This type of baldness is called seborrheic alopecia and is most common with very oily hair. Once the condition is corrected, healthy new hair will usually grow back. In the meantime, eating a balanced diet and cutting down on starches and animal fats will help considerably.

- Not combing your hair between settings can also lead to thinning hair and baldness. Usually this happens to women who go to a hairdresser weekly, have their hair set and then sprayed heavily to "hold" the set. At night when they go to bed, they carefully cover their hairdo with a net or cap, and the next morning—and for many mornings to follow—they comb just the ends of the hair. They never comb the entire head through, nor do they massage the scalp for fear of upsetting their hairdresser's "work of art." Unfortunately, as most of these women are in their later years, their circulation is often poor to begin with, and they may end up losing their hair.

Fortunately, all of these situations are fairly easy to correct. But if you take the proper precautions beforehand, it doesn't have to happen at all!

Choosing a New Hairstyle

Have you ever thought of changing your hairstyle and showing the world a "new you?" Great idea! I think that everyone, no matter how old, should do so whenever they feel the urge. But before you jump right in and choose "The Farrah" (made famous by Farrah Fawcett in the original "Charlie's Angels" television series) or an "Oleda" (not so famous, but a standard shoulder-length cut that I love), or a short bob, there are certain things you should consider.

1. The texture of your hair is the most important factor in selecting a hairstyle. Baby-fine hair is difficult to get to look like "The Farrah." it simply will not hold up. Nor will coarse, curly hair work well in a bob. But, no matter what type of hair you have, there is a style that will look great and accentuate your best features. So, my first rule for choosing a new hairstyle is to analyze your hair and look for a style that will complement it. Here are some guidelines.

    -   Thin hair without body usually needs a blunt, rather than layered cut.

    -   Medium to thick hair works best with a long style.

    -   If your hair doesn't take curl well and you don't want a permanent, wear it long and straight, or short enough so that you won't need to set it.

    -   The best style for coarse, curly hair is one that takes the curl into consideration, instead of fighting it. (You can use a conditioner to help soften it.)

    -   If you have baby-fine, straight hair, use a body building product after shampooing, no matter what hairstyle you have.

2. The second most important factor in my opinion is proportion—and I'm not just talking about the proportions of your face, but the entire shape of your figure from the top of your head to the tip of your toes.

    How many times have you seen a hairstyle that looked perfect on a woman—until she stood up? A long, bushy mane of hair will dwarf a small petite figure. Similarly, a sleek, sophisticated, but close-cropped head will look small and unbalanced on a very tall, overweight body.

    So, I suggest that you do this: Put on a bathing suit or leotard—anything that accurately conveys the proportions of your head and body. Slick your hair back and look at yourself in a full-length mirror. Are you short or tall? Full-figured or slim? Wide or narrow in the shoulders? High or low-waisted? Do you have a long body with short legs or vice versa? Then choose a hairstyle that helps create the illusion of a "more perfect" body.

- A soft, full hairdo tends to flatter a full figure because it balances the body and draws attention to the face.

- A triangular-shaped style (smaller at the crown, fuller at the bottom) can add height visually to a small woman by making the neck appear longer and drawing attention upward to the face.

- Longer hair on a tall woman—anywhere from the top of her shoulders to the middle of her back—will tend to "cut" the effect of height, whereas short, flattened hair will give the appearance of a small, sleek head and only emphasizes it. Long hair will also flatter a slim, shorter woman if she is not overweight.

- Big-boned women with wide hips and shoulders should wear a short, full haircut with upturned ends that will bring the eye up to the face and balance the strong horizontal lines of the body.

- A heavy-set woman with a short neck should wear her hair mid-neck or above and choose a hairstyle with a smooth, oval, overall shape. Long hair will give her the appearance of having no neck.

- A woman with a square, heavy-set face should choose a soft, curvy hairstyle that brings hair onto the face somewhat. This will "cut into" the face visually, breaking the square line.

- A pear-shaped face—wide at the bottom and narrow at the top— needs a hairstyle that slightly covers the cheeks.

- Thin, sharp facial features will look softer if surrounded with the touch of a curvy, rounded hairdo.

- Wide cheekbones look slimmer with a hairstyle that falls inward and slightly covers the sides of the face.

- Soft bangs are a smart choice to camouflage a very low or a very high forehead.

- A woman with a long, slender neck can wear long, full styles.

- A double chin is less noticeable when the hair comes forward on the face, rather than being swept tightly back.

3. The third most important factor is your lifestyle. How many times a week do you style your hair? Do you enjoy styling and experimenting with your hair? Or do you just want to set it and forget it until the next washing?

The point is this: If the care and maintenance of your new style takes more time than you're willing to give it, forget it. You'll just be miserable trying to keep up with its demands. So, take a good look at the way you live. Are you a career girl, a stay-at-home mom or a working mother? Do you have time for yourself each week, or are your hours filled with the demands of others? Are you the outdoor or indoor type? Do you engage in competitive sports or prefer more sedentary hobbies?

The answers to these questions will give you an idea as to which hairstyle you can best live with—a simple, basic or more elaborate one—and be happy with for as long as you choose to keep it. Don't forget you can always change it later.

COLORING YOUR HAIR

Since the beginning of time, women have been changing the color of their hair. In ancient Egypt, henna, a reddish-orange shade obtained from a shrub, was all the rage. Indigo, with its bluish tint, was a close runner-up, followed by sage, saffron, mixed alum, black sulphur and honey. Surprisingly, henna is once again very popular, but in a more sophisticated form.

Hair coloring has come a long way since ancient times, and many women are deciding that they don't want to be "type-cast" with the color they were born with. In fact, some 1.5 million American women go blond each year. Others spend more than $250 million annually to enrich their own, natural color.

I made my decision 52 years ago, and have never regretted it. I chose blond because that's the way I felt, instead of the medium-dark brown hair nature had given me. But there are dozens of other shades of red, brown or black that are not only beautiful, but may be more flattering to you than the color you are wearing now. On the other hand, don't feel that you have to change your hair color if you like it natural—that can be beautiful, too.

If you decide to make a change, you should not be afraid do so yourself at home. Gone are the days when hair coloring was unpredictable and only safe in the hands of a professional.

In deciding on your new hair color, it's a good idea to try on a wig in the particular shade that interests you. Try it on under all lighting conditions. And please keep in mind that, if you're going to change your hair color radically, you may have to change the color of your makeup and even some wardrobe, too. For example, if you're planning to change from medium brown to light blond, avoid orange-red lipsticks—they'll probably clash with your new hair color.

Once you've made up your mind and settled on a color, select your method carefully. Follow the instructions on the package step by step. For instance, most directions call for 2 important tests before you start to color your hair: the patch test for allergic reactions to the chemicals in the coloring, and the strand test to check how the product and shade will work on your individual hair. Don't skip them; they're very important to the success of the whole project.

Also keep in mind that you don't have to bleach or dye your entire head to achieve a color change. Frosting, tipping and streaking will help you achieve a lightened color without the drastic change of a complete makeover. And since they do not give a solid, all-over color, they require less touching up.

Basically, there are three kinds of hair coloring: temporary, semi-permanent and permanent.

1. **Temporary hair coloring.** Usually called "rinses" or "highlighting shampoos," these only last until your next shampoo. They don't actually lighten hair color, because they contain no bleaching agents. But they will add highlights and make subtle changes, since they coat the outside of the hair shaft. A rinse won't cover gray, but it will blend it in by adding a little color

to it. It can also eliminate the yellowish cast from white or gray hair. On hair that's already been chemically treated, it can revive color that has faded from permanent waving, sun or chlorine.

2. **Semi-permanent hair coloring.** These are gentle, penetrating colors and last from 3 to 5 shampoos. Again, they will not lighten hair because they contain no bleaching agents, but they will cover gray better, add highlights to natural hair or deepen your natural color. They not only coat the hair shaft, but they also gently penetrate its surface. Semi-permanent hair colors come either in lotions or aerosols. Lotions are more concentrated, work faster and make a stronger color difference. Aerosols are more diluted and have gentler effects. Both kinds, however, have conditioners added to give extra sheen along with extra color.

3. **Permanent hair coloring.** This is divided into 2 categories: one-step and two-step.

   1. **One-step hair coloring** is permanent, but can make the hair only a shade or 2 lighter. The hair must be touched up at the roots as it grows out. With one-step hair coloring you can brighten or darken natural hair color since it actually penetrates the hair shaft. It will also cover gray hair.

   2. **Two-step hair coloring** is precisely that: the first step completely bleaches the natural color from the hair shaft, and the second step puts the desired color back in. This method is used to become a medium to pale blonde or to frost, tip or streak. Depending on your lifestyle and how fast or slow your hair grows, you may need to touch up every 2 to 3 weeks to look your best. When modeling I had to touch up about every 10 days.

I am a two-step blonde, and although it requires a little extra work to stay that way, I feel that for me it's well worth it. Actually, by now I have it down to a science, so it takes very little time. I have the best of both worlds—I look like a blonde but think like a brunette!

Here are a few hints in order to get the most from your hair coloring.

- Apply hair coloring to dry hair. There is no need to pre-shampoo unless there is a heavy buildup of hair spray. If you do shampoo, be sure to dry your hair well. You'll get a better hair color that way.

- If you have a lot of gray, apply color to those areas first. Re-apply mixture all over head; follow regular instructions.

- Wait at least a week before coloring if you've just had a permanent wave or straightening.

- If any color solution gets into your eyes, rinse instantly with cool water.

- If mixture drips onto skin, to avoid staining or any irritation, rinse at once with lukewarm water. If it drips on clothing, wash the spot out immediately with soap and water.

- Color-treated hair needs special treatment because it's more vulnerable than other hair to drying, breakage and split ends.

- Make sure that you use a conditioner after every shampoo.

- Beware of strong sun, too-stiff setting lotions and hair sprays. Try to wear a scarf or hat when out in the sun for long periods of time.

TEASING HAIR

Unlike some other hair experts, I'm not against teasing the hair—if it's done right. I'm not advocating the kind of teasing that made beehive hairdos the rage in the 60's, but in moderation it can come in very handy to add height or give shape to an otherwise loose and swingy hairstyle. Here's how:

- Always use a comb, not a brush, to tease. The brush tangles too much of the hair at one time and makes it difficult to control the shape.

- Choose the area of the hair you wish to tease and, taking one section at a time, gently backcomb with smooth, slow, short strokes. I've seen women grab big chunks of their hair and rapidly "chop" away with fast, short movements. This approach can damage hair, causing breakage when you force the comb through the tangles. It can also result in a lumpy or clumpy look. Comb tangles out gently starting from the bottom up.

- Never tug or pull your hair with a comb or brush to remove the tangles. Instead, start at the edge and gently and slowly remove the outer tangles first. Then, work your way to the inside of the tangle. If this proves difficult, use your fingers to slowly pull the tangle apart.

- Don't sleep with teasing in your hair. Always brush your hair out completely before going to bed. Hair that is loose at night has a better chance to stay healthy. That goes for the scalp and hair follicles as well.

INSTANT FULLNESS TRICK

The natural fullness of your hair depends on the diameter and shape of each individual strand, as well as the total number of hairs on your head. Some people just have more hair than others, but you can control this to some degree. Feeding the follicles and roots properly will help new hair come in faster and stay in place longer, providing more fullness.

The quickest way to thicken your hair is to apply a hair body builder or a hair body thickener after washing it. After washing, I suggest using a light conditioner first. Rinse it off and towel dry before applying the instant thickener. Then set or style your hair as usual.

You can increase the width of each hair with a hair thickening product that contains water soluble panthenol. This "filler" travels into the cracks in the hair shaft, building it up, making it smoother and less porous. Although you still have the same number of hairs, they give the appearance of a fuller head of hair because their shafts are fatter.

A good haircut can also make you look as if you have more hair. However, you should follow these guidelines.

- For very straight hair, stick to a blunt or semi-blunt cut; the less layering the better.

- With curly hair, a good layered cut can release the hair's natural spring.

- With very fine hair worn too long, the weight of the hair will drag it down and give it a thin, scraggly look. Cut a little shorter, it can at least give the illusion of fullness and bulk.

One surefire way to add body to limp hair is to get a light permanent—one that does not make your hair curly. Today's permanents can be controlled to give you anything from Little Orphan Annie curls to "The Farrah" look. However, if you are giving yourself a home permanent, read the labels carefully and follow all instructions to the letter. If you're going to a hair salon, make sure the beautician gives you exactly what you want.

ADDITIONAL HAIR TIPS

- To give natural or colored hair that is starting to look faded a special "lift," mix the juice of half a lemon, 1/2 ounce of a mild shampoo, and 1 teaspoon of 3% medicinal peroxide. Shampoo into wet hair, leave for 2 to 5 minutes, rinse out, and see the difference!

- To bring out highlights in red or blond hair, rinse with cider vinegar. Then use the juice of half a lemon added to a glass of icy cold water for a final rinse.

- For exceptionally dry or dull hair, put a drop or 2 of rosemary oil in your palm. Run the bristles of your hairbrush through it and then whisk over your hair.

- The old notion that "more suds" means "more clean" is an old wives' tale. You can apply so much shampoo that it fails to rinse out properly, leaving a dull, filmy haze. So, use enough shampoo, but don't overdo it.

- Poor hair equipment can ruin hair. Throw out broken combs or too-hard brushes that scratch the scalp. Your comb should have wide spaces between the teeth, and rounded ends.

- To give clean, fresh hair that extra special touch, add a drop or 2 of your favorite cologne to one cup of cool water and use as a final rinse. Or, when hair is dry, hold a cologne bottle 6 to 8 inches from hair and give it a light spray.

AFTERTHOUGHTS

If anyone should have dull, dry hair and split ends, it's me! Not only have I colored my hair since I was 23 years old, I always bleach it first. So for 53 years I have "abused" my hair. But I have also provided the hair follicles with good nutrition, massaged my scalp regularly and used conditioners to help prevent damage. And one more thing—I have bleached, colored, conditioned, washed, set and also cut my hair myself. That way I have ensured that my hair was not over-bleached and that it always got cut the way I wanted!

PART 2: INSIDE

---

*The words "old age" are obsolete
if you take care of yourself.*

I'm not sure how it all came about, although, I do remember as a young teenager my father using the word "preventive" a lot. He made a decision to change his lifestyle in his early 40s. Until then, he had been overweight, tired and a cigarette smoker. When he developed a limp in one leg, he went to see a doctor who told him to "get a cane." That remark infuriated my father so much that he stomped out of the office, did his own research to find the cause, and began to take charge of his own health…and life. He stopped smoking, lost weight and built a homemade gym in the garage. Most evenings he took long walks after dinner. His limp disappeared and he stayed slim the rest of his life. I remember admiring his resourcefulness, and I believe that it marked the beginning of my own efforts to prevent health problems before they acted up…and then carried it further throughout my life.

As a model I studied other, more experienced models who had been in the business a long time. What did they know and do—and what did other people in the beauty and health and fashion business know—that kept them looking and feeling younger for their age than others?

When I was young I thought models were just born "that way." But stepping into New York City's high fashion world, I soon learned differently. Whatever natural beauty they possessed, "the look" came just as much from their inside glow and health. I watched them take care of themselves and found it fascinating that they paid as much attention to the things that affected them inside as what made them look good on the outside. There was no part of their body they were not concerned about. Nutrition, diet, exercise and proper sleeping habits were always on their minds, especially the ones that lasted in the business. I was 38 years old when I stopped modeling with Wilhelmina. At the time, I was one of the oldest still in the fashion world while others had moved on.

The main reason was that I followed in their and my father's footsteps, except that I practiced preventive care much more aggressively as it pertained to the health of my body both inside and out.

In this section, I will share with you some of the things I learned while taking care of my body from the inside that have enabled me to celebrate my 75th birthday with such great health and flexibility. I know that it was my father's stick-to-itiveness that inspired me. I'm hoping that, with what you have already read so far and what's coming now in these next chapters, I can similarly inspire you!

CHAPTER 6

FOOD, VITAMINS AND SUPPLEMENTS

Your health, beauty, energy and longevity depend on what you put into your body.

In the early- to mid-1900s, a 50-year-old person was considered old and usually looked it. Today, with the baby boomers leading the parade, people are learning there is a choice. For one thing, science is slowly winning the battle against many serious illnesses. Yet we cannot expect the medical profession to do it alone. Taking on the day-to-day responsibility ourselves ensures a flexible, healthy body with lots of energy and youthful skin and hair.

The human body consists of about 200 different types of cells, which all together number in the trillions, even in a small child. Some sources estimate that an average person has 50 to 100 trillion cells.

Your cells vary in size, but even the largest can only be seen through a microscope; and even though they're so very tiny, they're complex, made up of many parts.

Some glandular cells produce hormones or enzymes; some cells in your mouth produce saliva; cells in a woman's breasts produce milk; some in the pancreas produce insulin; and some in the lining of the lungs produce mucus. Red blood cells carry oxygen throughout the body, skin cells protect the body, bone cells make the skeleton, and nerve cells send messages around the body. Bacterial cells in your digestive system perform several important functions, such as synthesizing various vitamins, converting food into energy and building blocks for the body, and processing waste products.

Your cells are constantly renewing themselves. Your skin cells flaking off are part of that process. Within 3 or 4 months your total blood supply will be replaced. Internal organs take more time. Bone cells take the longest. This cell regeneration gets slower as each year rolls by, and that is what causes a person's body to look and feel older.

So how do we compensate for this natural slowing down of cell growth? Primarily by choosing to eat and not eat certain things—proper nutrition that may include supplements—as well as other healthy lifestyle activities, like exercise and getting proper rest.

The process of cell rejuvenation is not completely understood. Most theories hold that aging is caused by damage to our DNA over time. DNA is our genetic blueprint found in chromosomes within our cells' nuclei. Each time cells divide, the ends of the chromosomes, caps called telomeres, become a tiny bit shorter, until reproduction stops and the cell becomes senescent, meaning old. Senescent cells don't die; rather, they emit certain proteins that can harm other nearby cells and can contribute to cancer and aging.

However, as scientists continue to study this process, more and more is being understood about how we can sustain our cells in maintaining their vitality and extending their life cycles. One thing we have come to learn: A longer, healthier life depends on how you take care of your cells, and a great deal has to do with how you nourish them. You are what you eat—really![5]

> OUR CELLS ARE THE BUILDING BLOCKS OF THE ONLY BODY WE'LL EVER HAVE.

In order for your cells to function well, they need to be fed properly with a whole series of nutrients: macronutrients, which are proteins, carbohydrates and fats; and micronutrients, which are vitamins and minerals. It is possible to get these nutrients from the food you eat, and, in order to get them all, you need the proverbial "well-balanced" diet.

MACRONUTRIENTS: PROTEINS, CARBOHYDRATES AND FATS

Macronutrients in the food you eat provide the energy, in the form of calories, your body needs. They sustain growth and regulate metabolism and other bodily functions. They are required in large quantities.

CARBOHYDRATES

Carbohydrates are your main source of fuel, providing glucose—a kind of sugar—which your heart, central nervous system and kidneys need for their basic maintenance. Glucose is the only substance your brain uses for energy.

Simple carbohydrates are digested quickly. They contain refined sugars with few essential vitamins and minerals: fruit juice, yogurt, honey, molasses, sugar, candy, cake, soda pop, bread and pasta made with white flour and many packaged cereals.

Complex carbohydrates are larger molecules, so it takes longer for your body to break them down and use them. They provide the majority of essential vitamins and minerals you need, and they contain fiber to help your intestinal tract expel waste, and help lower cholesterol. Examples are oatmeal, bran, brown rice, brown bread, root vegetables, whole grain cereals, high fiber breakfast cereals, peas, beans, yams, lentils and corn.

Most mainstream nutritionists agree that 45 to 65% of our daily diet should be made up of carbohydrates. In order to achieve that, we should concentrate on fruits, vegetables, beans, seeds, nuts and whole grains. Cut down on starchy foods like pasta, white bread and potatoes.

I don't think highly of formal diets. They're boring, cumbersome and time consuming, and, for most people, too difficult to stay with. Even dieters who reach their goals most often revert to old diet habits and regain what they lost.

Years ago a publisher asked me to write a book about my diet. He figured I must know something special since I maintained the same weight year in and year out. I refused, because a diet book by me would have had only one page with three words: "Just eat less!"

Now, 30 years later, I still weigh the same—120 pounds. I eat everything, just less of it. My own practice and belief is with the mainstream. I believe in a balanced diet for my high-energy needs and, if my jeans start to get tight, I simply cut down on my calorie intake by eating smaller portions for a while.

PROTEINS

All our living cells, muscles, organs, and almost all our fluids have proteins as their main component. Proteins are complex formations and various combinations of 20 amino acids. Half of them can be produced by our body, but the other 10, which are called essential amino acids, can only be obtained by eating the right foods. Poultry, fish, wheat germ, beans and dairy products all contain these essential amino acids.

Amino acids make up 75% of the human body, after removing water and fat, and they are crucial to nearly every bodily function. Every chemical reaction that takes place in your body depends on amino acids and the proteins that they build. Without proteins, life would be impossible.

FATS

Fat is bad for you. Fat is good for you. I hear you saying, "Well, Oleda, make up your mind. Which is it?" Both! Fat, like protein, is necessary for a healthy body. We need fats to help nutrient absorption, nerve transmission and the maintenance of our cell membranes. Some fats promote those functions while others increase our risk of disease.

Good fats come in 2 versions:

- Monosaturated fats are found in peanuts, walnuts, almonds, pistachios, avocado, canola oil and olive oil.

- Polyunsaturated fats are found in seafood, like salmon and fish oil, soy, safflower oil and sunflower oil.

Bad fats also come in 2 versions:

- Saturated fats, high in cholesterol, are mainly found in meat, dairy, eggs, coconut oil and palm oil.

- Trans fats, by far the worst, are created by treating processed foods to provide longer shelf life. They're found in many commercially packaged foods, commercially fried food, other packaged snacks such as microwaved popcorn, as well as in vegetable shortening and hard stick margarine.

Can you avoid bad fats completely? No, but you can certainly minimize your intake of them.

Want to lose weight? There is only one good way: Burn more calories than you take in on a daily basis through a program of a healthy, balanced diet and exercise. Consider this: Carbohydrates contain 4 calories per gram. Proteins contain 4 calories per gram. Fats, good or bad, contain 9 calories per gram.

Do the math.

And here's another fact: Alcohol contains 7 calories per gram, and these are so called "empty" calories because alcohol contains no nutrients...none whatsoever!

MICRONUTRIENTS: VITAMINS AND MINERALS

VITAMINS

Vitamins are small molecules your body needs—all those many trillions of cells—in order to work; minerals help them do their job.

There are 2 basic types of vitamins:

- Water soluble: Vitamins B1 (thiamine), B2 (riboflavin), B3 (niacin), B5 (pantothenic acid), B6 (pyridoxin), B12 (cyanocobalamin), and folic acid, vitamin C (ascorbic acid) and biotin. The water soluble vitamins don't stay around long. Once they've done their job traveling through your bloodstream, the excess is eliminated with your urine. Therefore, they have to be replaced every day.

- Fat soluble: Vitamins A, D, E and K. These vitamins last from a few days up to 6 months and only get used when your body tells them they're needed.

MINERALS

Unlike organic substances like vitamins, minerals are inorganic elements that come from the soil and water. They are essential for processes such as muscle contractions, blood clotting and nerve reactions. For example, eating a diet rich in iron can help your hemoglobin level (the protein in red blood cells that stores the oxygen) stay high enough for all the cells in your body to get the oxygen they need to function properly. When our bodies don't get enough minerals, they draw from those stored in the liver, muscles and even bones. creating an imbalance and depletion in the system

There are 2 types of minerals:

- Major minerals, of which your body requires more than 100 milligrams per day, are sodium chloride, potassium, calcium, phosphorus, magnesium, manganese and sulphur.

■ Trace minerals, of which your body needs less than 100 milligrams per day, are iron, zinc, copper, selenium, iodine, fluorine and chromium.

Because your body cannot manufacture minerals, you have to obtain them from the food you eat.

What If You Don't Get Sufficient Vitamins and Minerals from the Food You Eat?

The vitamin and supplements industry is a multi-billion-dollar business in the United States, eager to sell as many products as possible. Although many healthy people can get their full complement of vitamins and minerals from their diets, many people feel they need supplements. You must remember that the older you get, the less your body can absorb from food, so supplements are certainly recommended.

Be careful, though; it is possible to overdose. Fat soluble vitamins or minerals, which are stored in the body, are more difficult to excrete and can build up in your system to levels where they could cause problems.

If you're on a weight loss program, skipping meals, or if you're pregnant or elderly, you may need to use vitamins and supplements. Check with your doctor or a registered dietician. They can help you design a proper diet that may or may not include supplements.

I'm on the go so much at age 75, I know I don't always get the chance to sit down to proper meals, so I take 4 supplements every day:

■ an all-purpose vitamin capsule that includes major and trace minerals

■ a vegetable and fruit concentrate made up of 12 fruits and vegetables (I take the powder form at home and capsule when traveling)

■ an aloe vera juice concentrate (or aloe vera concentrate capsule when I travel)

■ a B-complex vitamin which I have been taking for over 40 years.

The last time I had my nutrition levels checked, my doctor had blood samples sent to a special laboratory where they performed FIA (Functional Intracellular Analysis), a procedure that measures nutrient levels. The results of my test indicated that I was within the proper spectrum on everything, but my doctor suggested some slight alterations in my diet and some temporary supplementation in order to optimize my nutrition levels. I strongly suggest you check with your doctor about doing such testing periodically for yourself.

Note: *Whenever considering supplements, it is important to go over any medications you may be taking with your physician or pharmacist to avoid any adverse interactions. Even good nutrients can cause some medications to not work as prescribed or possibly not work at all.*

Water—an Important Health Aid

Water qualifies as a nutrient—it contains trace minerals—but its importance in your health is second only to the air you breathe. Your body's total makeup is 67% water. It is involved in your digestion, absorption, circulation and elimination. Keeping your body hydrated is essential for timely and efficient functioning of these processes. Simply put, all of your body functions require water.

Dehydration is one of the most common causes of fatigue. Almost 2/3 of Americans are mildly or chronically dehydrated. I always keep a bottle of water close by while I'm writing or in the art studio where I paint. I also put a bottle of water next to my husband sometimes to encourage his water intake. Keeping a bottle close by encourages you to drink more.

Water helps maintain a normal body temperature and is essential for carrying waste material from the body, including through the pores of your skin. Therefore, it is necessary to replace the water that is continually lost through sweat and elimination.

There are many other benefits of water: improved skin tone; appetite regulation; increased metabolism; greater energy; reduced cholesterol; blood pressure control. Water reduces headaches, relieves joint pain and decreases the risk of developing kidney stones.

Drink at least 8 glasses of water every day. Remember the body can survive without food for about 5 weeks, but only 5 days without water.

The Dangers of Soda Pop

Some people drink soda as if it were water. Sure, there's lots of water in them but, with all the other "stuff" they contain, drinking a lot of it is a surefire way to age faster. If

I drink 2 sodas a year, that would be a lot for me! It might be that knowing how bad it is for your health, looks and, yes, even life, I don't even like the taste of it.

Sodas contain an alarming amount of sugar, empty calories and harmful additives. There's phosphoric acid, caffeine and, in diet sodas, aspartame, artificial coloring, and sulphites, none of which have nutritional value. Studies have linked soda to osteoporosis, obesity, tooth decay and heart disease.

The average American drinks an estimated 56 gallons of soft drinks each year. I hope you or your children are not contributing to that statistic.

My only recommendation: Stay away from it. Wait...I do have another recommendation: Keep your kids away from it, too!

HELP FOR THE BLOATED STOMACH

One of the more common health and beauty problems women ask me about is "bloated stomach." This is characterized by a swollen abdomen, caused by an expansion of the lower intestine (not the stomach). It doesn't look good, and it gives you an uncomfortable feeling. Most of the time, bloated stomach is a result of irregular digestion that produces a higher than normal rate of gas. There are many causes, but the primary ones are eating too fast, eating too much, eating foods you can't tolerate, having irregular movements, the habit of swallowing air, lactose intolerance, irritable bowel syndrome and partial bowel obstruction.

Eating a lot late at night, without giving yourself at least three hours before lying down in bed, can also result in a bloated stomach. You might even notice it if you begin a health diet, because of the sudden increase in fiber from vegetables, fruits and beans. (If that happens, cut down on those foods and introduce them into your diet more gradually.)

If you've tried some lifestyle changes, reducing the more common causes listed above, check with your doctor to make sure there's no medical condition causing excessive gas. After that, experiment with cutting back on or completely eliminating typical gas-producing foods. These include beans, cabbage, onions, cauliflower, broccoli, apples, peaches, pears, prunes, corn, oats, potatoes, wheat and milk products. Foods that produce minimal gas include rice, bananas, citrus, grapes, meat, eggs, peanut butter, non-carbonated beverages, and yogurt made with live bacteria.

SPECIAL ENZYMES FOR DIGESTION CAN HELP

It's no secret that for many it becomes harder to enjoy a meal without suffering from some type of digestive discomfort. Every 10 years of life, the pancreas produces fewer digestive enzymes. In addition, our modern diets are largely devoid of natural plant enzymes. An overall lack of enzymes causes the body to work harder, putting a strain on our internal organs and digestive system.

Knowing what to eat can help you build up enzymes and lead to creating a more comfortable, flatter stomach. Spices such as ginger root, fennel seeds and clove powder aid digestion. Other things that might be helpful include simethicone, an anti-gas product, peppermint leaf extract and acid stable protease.

FREE RADICALS AND ANTIOXIDANTS

Some of the more damaging molecules in your body, responsible for aging, tissue damage and disease, are free radicals.

Their name comes from the fact that they have lost an electron due to oxidation and, as they are looking to replace it, steal one from another molecule, causing a chain reaction of instability and damage. They are a natural by-product of metabolism, but can be built up to excess as a result of stress, cigarettes, ultraviolet rays of the sun, toxic chemicals from pollution and pesticides in foods.

Antioxidants neutralize these destructive molecules by giving them one of their own electrons, ending the chain reaction. The antioxidant nutrients themselves don't become free radicals because they are stable in either form. Antioxidants help prevent the cell and tissue damage that causes aging and disease.

One of the most noticeable areas of free radical damage is the skin. Antioxidants alone cannot eliminate wrinkles or other effects of aging but, combined with a good skin care regimen, they will go a long way toward minimizing the negative effects.

Most nutritionists suggest you eat 5 cups of fruits and vegetables per day. The more colorful the fruit or vegetable, the more benefits you will derive. The best-known antioxidants are vitamins C and E, alpha- and beta-carotene, lycopene, lutein and ze-axanthin.

Eating the fruits and vegetables to get the antioxidants you need every day might not be possible. You might not have the time, inclination or the taste for them. In that case, adding supplements like vitamins A, C and E to your daily intake is a way to ensure you are getting the minimum daily requirement, and at the same time guarding against possible weight gain. One way or another, your body must have antioxidants to neutralize free radicals and reduce the age damage they cause.

VITAMIN C is found in oranges, grapefruit, broccoli, leafy vegetables, tomatoes, peppers, cantaloupe and strawberries.

VITAMIN E is found in vegetable oils, walnuts, peanuts, almonds, seeds, olives, avocado and liver.

ALPHA- and BETA-CAROTENE is found in vegetable oil, green leafy vegetables and nuts.

LYCOPENE, LUTEIN and ZEAXANTHIN. Lycopene is found in tomatoes and other red fruits and vegetables. Good sources for lutein and zeaxanthin are eggs, spinach, kale, brussels sprouts, broccoli and kiwi fruits.

Three Exceptional Nutrition Sources

Prunes

Prunes contain twice the antioxidants of the next best single food item—raisins. When buying prunes, the package should be sealed well to ensure moistness—try vacuum-packed containers. You can keep prunes at home for snacks and take them with you anywhere. Keep sealed and dry and they will last for months.

You might like to get out your cookbook and look for a good dessert recipe. *The Joy of Cooking* has a delicious prune compote recipe. You can also mix pureed prunes when baking and add them to meat dishes.

Blueberries

Low in calories and high in antioxidants and fiber, blueberries help protect the heart by reducing cholesterol, and may help reduce cardiac inflammation. Studies also suggest that eating blueberries may help fight cancer and diabetes, reduce the risk of stroke, and improve cognition. One cup of blueberries contains 15% of your daily vitamin C requirement and 14% of daily dietary fiber (see Oleda's personal health drink below for blueberry recipe).

Aloe Vera

The aloe vera plant consists of three main parts: the leaves, the sap and the gel. For best results, it is important that these elements interact, although the sap is considered the most active ingredient. I take aloe vera juice every day and would not want to be without it.

Aloe vera is available in capsules or in liquid concentrate for mixing in juice. Used topically, it is one of the best skin conditioners in the world. Look for creams and lotions with aloe vera as the first listed ingredient.

It also contains anti-inflammatory fatty acids, which is why it is an effective treatment for burns, cuts and abrasions. If you have an aloe plant in your yard, just cut a piece off and place the sap on the burn or cut. Otherwise use an aloe cream

Aloe vera is just as beneficial for the inside of your body. It helps in cell protection, cellular oxygenation, and contains antioxidants, as well as anti-viral, anti-bacterial, and anti-fungal aids. It is thought to help keep the intestinal tract (lining) cleaner. The plant further produces antiseptics that can control mold, bacteria, fungus and viruses. Therefore, it can reduce or eliminate many internal and external infections.

Don't buy cheap aloe products found in supermarkets or drugstores. Aloe vera that will best benefit your health is greenhouse-grown without insecticides. It should be processed at temperatures that do not destroy the biological activity of the plant. You'll find such aloe in a health-oriented store or on my website at www.oleda.com.

Oleda's Personal Health Drink

No time to shop or cook? Need energy in a hurry? Try my personal energy/nutritional-easy-to-make-all-in-one-container meal. I have it for lunch 4 or 5 times a week. It's filling, delicious and very healthy. Drink one of these several times a week and you'll be giving the cells in your body a real boost.

Here's what you need:

- A blender
- Large container of vanilla yogurt (32 oz.)
- 2 to 3 cups of blueberries
- 1 to 1½ cups of strawberries (I keep both berries in the freezer at all times)
- 1 or 2 bananas (if you don't have them, it's just as good without them)
- Honey

Here's what you do:

- Put defrosted blueberries and strawberries into blender.
- Add cut banana in large pieces and drop in blender.
- Put about half of the container of yogurt in blender to start.
- Mix well, then add more yogurt, leaving room for honey.
- Sweeten to taste (I like mine on the sweet side).
- Turn blender to "liquefy" or "puree" for best results.
- Pour one glass of health drink for yourself now and add any remaining yogurt to what's left in the blender. Mix again.

This will produce 4 to 5 glasses of delicious, fortifying drink. Have one glass now. Put a plastic sandwich bag over the rest. Refrigerated, it will last for several days.

AFTERTHOUGHTS

There's so much more to know, and so I encourage you to take it further and keep learning. For now, though, just remember, you truly are what you eat. I hope you believe that now. Carbohydrates, proteins, fats, vitamins, amino acids, water and antioxidants: We need them all, and they're all interactive.

And don't be confused by all the combinations of different foods that are the sources of all these nutrients. Notice how overlapping all those groups are. Just follow the Mayo Clinic's recommendation of 50% carbohydrates, 25% proteins and 25% fats daily. Try to concentrate on the complex carbs and good fats and, if your lifestyle prevents you from getting a proper diet daily, get to your vitamin store for some good supplements. That's what I do.

CHAPTER 7

KNOW YOUR HORMONE LEVELS

For an agile body, youthful skin, hair and bones, your hormones need to be in balance.

After my last bone density test my doctor came into the room with the results. He looked rather puzzled as he stared at the paper. I got nervous and asked him if there was a problem. He looked at me strangely, as if I were some alien creature and said, "You have the bone density of a 23-year-old." Needless to say, I was delighted. I have been on Hormone Replacement Therapy (HRT) for about 25 years and swear by it.

There has been some controversy over how good or bad HRT is for your body, and I'll get to that. But first, let's talk about what it is and why I believe it to be one of the important weapons in the anti-aging arsenal.

HORMONE BASICS

Hormones are basically messengers that allow cells to communicate with each other and trigger certain functions. In women the hormones estrogen and progesterone are produced in the ovaries, along with other hormones, including small amounts of the male hormone, testosterone. They normally increase and decrease according to your monthly reproductive cycle.

Estrogen builds up the lining of the uterus, stimulates breast tissue and thickens the vaginal wall, but it affects other parts of your body as well, including every organ. It also plays an important role in bone building.

Progesterone prepares the uterine lining for egg implantation and has other important effects on many of the tissues sensitive to estrogen.

Testosterone plays a role in stimulating sexual desire, generating energy and developing muscle mass.

Proper balance is very important for your entire body. The cells in the vagina, bladder, breasts, skin, bones, arteries, heart, liver and brain all contain estrogen receptors, and require the hormone to stimulate them for normal cell function.

Stress, body weight, time of day, time of the month and any medications you take can all cause temporary changes in your hormone levels. But what really throws them out of balance for good is menopause. During that time, your ovaries stop producing eggs, and estrogen and progesterone production tapers off, although many women are already generating less progesterone by their late 30s. It is the fluctuations in estrogen and, later, the lack of it, that are the primary cause of the discomforts and health concerns that are associated with menopause.

The symptoms—hot flashes and vaginal dryness—can be treated by replacing estrogen and progesterone after menopause. However, the major benefits of HRT are prevention of osteoperosis (the weakening of bones) and protection against heart disease.

Replacing estrogen in particular can help prevent slow bone loss, increase bone density and aid in the absorption of calcium, which gives bones strength.

Women are more prone to cardiovascular disease after menopause because the blood vessels leading to their hearts become narrowed. HRT helps reduce bad cholesterol that can build up inside the blood vessels while increasing good cholesterol, thereby helping to keep the arteries clear.

CONTROVERSIES AND MYTHS

There has been some controversy about whether HRT is good or harmful for your body. Many people believe, on little credible evidence, that it causes cancer. I have no ax to grind in the matter. I just want to suggest that women who are currently on or considering going on estrogen/progesterone replacement therapy discuss the issues involved with their doctor, rather than form conclusions based on information in sensationalized and misleading news media reports.

In 2002, a major 5-year study on HRT was abruptly halted by federal researchers of the Women's Health Initiative (WHI), because they said they detected an increased risk of health problems. Alarming stories about this appeared in all the news media.

At the time, I stated my belief that this was another case of reporting dangers disproportionate to reality As it turned out, the study was limited to older women who were well past their menopausal years. Two years later, a review of other studies of younger women who began HRT before turning 60 revealed that HRT actually reduced the risk of dying from any cause by 39% compared to women who did not undergo HRT at all.[6, 7] Most of those studies were conducted between 1990 and 2002. Where were these reports about younger women in 2002, when the controversy was raging?

Then, in 2006, findings published in the Journal of Women's Health showed that women who began HRT shortly after entering menopause had a 30% lower risk for heart disease than women who did not. A fresh analysis of the WHI data, published in the Archives of Internal Medicine, suggested that health concerns about HRT may have been overstated. Even the WHI then advised women to consult their doctor about HRT.

> AT AGE 75, I HAVE NO SIGN OF OSTEOPOROSIS, AND MY BONES ARE AS DENSE AS THOSE OF SOMEONE 50 YEARS YOUNGER THAN ME!

In August 2008, one of the world's longest and largest trials of hormone replacement therapy found that postmenopausal women on HRT gain significant improvements in quality of life. The results of the latest study by the WISDOM (women's international study of long-duration oestrogen after menopause) research team can be found on the British Medical Journal website at www.bmj.com.[8, 9, 10]

Despite these studies, HRT remains controversial. In 2008, a study conducted in New York indicated a possible link between HRT and breast cancer in some women.

But based on my own HRT experience of nearly 25 years and all the positive findings over the last 18 years, I urge anyone having menopausal or pre-menopausal problems to discuss the possibility of HRT with a competent doctor.

If you would like to try HRT, check with your doctor to see if you're a candidate—not everyone is—but make sure he or she understands the studies. Some doctors dismiss HRT because they don't know enough about it and don't want to bother with it. Others just want to play it safe (for themselves), but that may not be the best answer for you.

For me the benefits have outweighed the supposed negatives for nearly a quarter century. At age 75, I have no sign of osteoporosis, and my bones are as dense as those of someone 50 years younger than me! I believe that the HRT I've been on—along with the proper diet, supplements and exercise—is the reason for my strong bones and agile body, not to mention my youthful-looking skin.

Nutrition for Hormones

One way to aid hormone development is to eat foods that encourage their production, in partiular phytoestrogens, also known as plant estrogens. These estrogen-like compounds are found in soybeans, tofu, miso, flaxseeds, pomegranates and dates. Japanese women who eat these foods regularly are known to experience far fewer symptoms of menopause than women in the United States or Europe.

Afterthoughts

Recently, one of the newsletters sent by my company to its database of opted-in recipients dealt with the subject of HRT and noted essentially the same thing I've written in this chapter. One of the people who received the newsletter was an acquaintance who had successfully fought a bout with breast cancer over the previous 12 or 14 months. It happened that she and her husband came into a local restaurant while my husband and I were dining there with friends. As soon as she spotted me, before allowing herself to be seated, she rushed over to our table and loudly proclaimed her displeasure over the newsletter. She said it was HRT that caused her cancer, and I should not be advising women to take it. I tried to explain that my advice is not to automatically go on HRT, but, rather, to consult a competent doctor about it to see if you're a candidate, consider all the pros and cons, and then make an informed decision. I could not get that point across to her that evening, but I'm including this story here in order to reiterate 2 things: First, that HRT has been a godsend for me and many other women. And second, find a well-versed gynecologist who can properly advise you without influence from the "hysterical" media.

CHAPTER 8

WEIGHT

Weight may be the single most important factor for your beauty, health and longevity.

No, I don't think everyone has to be "thin," but I do believe everyone should work to be healthy and keep their weight within the proper limits for their height and body type. Remember, it's how you take care of the cells in your body, regardless of your age, that will determine your future health, beauty and longevity.

When considering how much you should weigh, you need to consider your body type, height and the size of your bones. Let's say a small-boned woman weighs 120 pounds. A woman of the same height with a medium frame might weigh 130 pounds, while someone with a large frame could top 140 pounds or more and still be within proper weight standards. In addition, you might be a person with heavier muscles. Take a look at yourself in the mirror, figure out what your weight should be (maybe with the help of your doctor) and then, if you need to, set your goal and start working toward it right away.

OBESITY—AN EPIDEMIC

Obesity among adults in the United States has increased about 50% per decade since 1980. Research has shown that the life expectancy of people who are severely obese—with a body mass index (BMI) greater than 45—is up to 20 years lower than people who are not overweight.[11] (BMI measures the relationship between a person's weight and height. A person 5' 5" inches tall, weighing 180 pounds has a BMI of 30, and is considered to have reached obesity.)

Research suggests that obesity causes about 300,000 deaths in the U.S. every year from various illnesses.[12] Here's why: The engorged fat cells in an obese person produce toxic chemicals that injure blood vessels, raise cholesterol, and cause high blood pressure, diabetes, metabolic syndrome, strokes, cancer and infertility. Moreover, when all the fat cells are filled up, they start producing new chemicals circulating in the bloodstream and they create new fat cells that are even more dangerous.

Studies indicate that of the 570,000 cancer deaths expected in the U.S. annually, obesity and poor nutrition are linked to 190,000 of them, which is about the same number of cancer deaths from smoking.

The New England Journal of Medicine reported on a 16-year study of 57,145 cancer deaths among a group of 900,000 people. None of the participants had cancer when they enrolled in the study. It was found that 20% of all cancer deaths among women and 14% among men were associated with being overweight. For almost all cancers, the risk of death increased in direct proportion to body mass. Among women, the heaviest of them in the study were 62% more likely to die of cancer than women of normal weight.

Moreover, these cancer deaths were not confined to malignancies with previously known links to excess body weight, such as breast and colorectal cancers. Many cancers not previously associated with obesity were identified as being caused by obesity, including stomach cancer and prostate cancer, cancers of the cervix, ovary, liver, pancreas, and multiple myeloma and non-Hodgkin's lymphoma.

In addition to shortening one's life span, obesity prevents us from looking our best, often lowers our self-esteem and frequently denies happy day-to-day living.

Take your face, for example. As a person gains too much weight, facial tissue and skin become thicker and heavier, too. The facial muscles must carry the additional weight, which, over time, stretches the muscles downward and brings the skin and tissue along with it. The skin becomes droopy and the face becomes older-looking before its time. Deep lines set in. That's one reason there are so many facelifts "needed" today.

I am 5' 8" tall and have small bones. I have weighed between 119 pounds and 123 pounds all my adult life (except when I was pregnant). My weight-to-height ratio is a bit unusual because my muscles are not heavy and I stay a little on the thin side on purpose.

I'm energetic and very flexible. I have never been on a "formal" diet and eat everything I have a taste for, just not a lot of it. As I mentioned before, if I feel my favorite pair of jeans getting a bit tight, I reduce my calorie intake a little and rev up the treadmill to a faster walking speed until my jeans once again fit the way I want them to. This means that I pay close attention to my eating habits and daily nutrition.

My recommendation: Get your weight to where you want it; don't let it get out of hand. Life will be much simpler that way.

OBESITY AND CHILDREN

If you're a parent, you have the power and responsibility to control your child's diet. We are all born with a specific number of fat cells. As your children grow and mature, they continue to add fat cells up to a certain age. Studies indicate that children who eat more food accumulate more cells. Obese children can have 2 to 5 times more fat cells than a child of proper weight. Obese children will grow up to become obese adults.

When children reach adolescence, the number of fat cells will be fixed in their bodies throughout life. That means obese children will have a body that is programmed to store fat. As a result it will be more difficult for them to lose weight and keep it off.

Children who were fortunate enough to be brought up with a healthy diet and regular physical activity will have fewer fat cells. They are likely to remain slender, and when they put on a few extra pounds, they will have an easier time losing them.

So, if you want to give your children a leg up in the weight department, it's very important to instill good eating habits from the beginning and to get them to be active outdoors, not just sitting around playing video games or watching TV all day.

If you are an overweight parent, you can change your children's so called "heredity," which is often bad habits passed down from one generation to the next. Tell them you know you are overweight and don't want it to happen to them. And tell them why.

BROWN FAT VS. WHITE FAT

We've been taught that fat is bad, but the truth is, some fat is very healthy for us! Take a look at 2 different types of fat: brown and white:

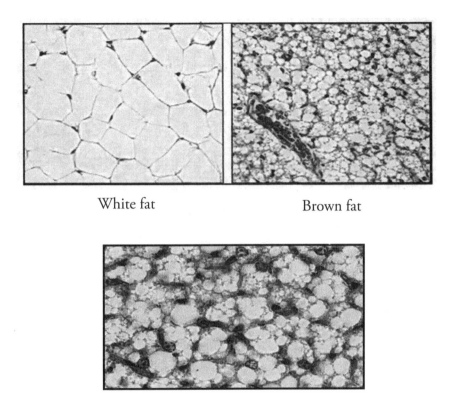

White fat   Brown fat

Enlarged diagram of brown fat

Brown fat feels and looks firmer and healthier than white fat. It has a considerable volume of cytoplasm (fluid that is critical to the cells' survival), contains lipid droplets (fatty acid) of varying size, and has an abundance of blood-filled capillaries. The cell nuclei are round and almost centrally located. White fat (it is actually yellowish in color), on the other hand, has a scant ring of cytoplasm surrounding a single large lipid droplet. The cell nuclei are flattened and eccentric within the cell. This is soft, unhealthy fat, which stores up calories and stubbornly accumulates around waistlines, hips, thighs and buttocks.

HOW THE TWO FATS INTERRELATE

Is all white fat bad? No. Hibernating animals, for example, store huge amounts of white fat in anticipation of winter to keep them warm, using a bodily process called thermogenesis, which produces heat. Simply put, it is brown fat consuming white fat.

Brown fat when stimulated burns stored white fat, converting calories to heat and energy. According to one scientific study, 3 ounces of brown fat would be enough, if maximally stimulated, to burn up 400 to 500 calories per day. So, a little bit can go a long way.

There is an abundance of blood-filled capillaries and variable sizes of lipid droplets in good brown fat. But converting your body from soft white fat to firm brown fat is something only you can do. You can help thermogenesis along by increasing your metabolic rate, which can be activated by a few different mechanisms, including nutrition, exercise and supplements.

HERBALS FOR FAT BURNING

Thermogenesis (good brown fat comsuming bad white fat) can be directly stimulated by certain herbs. But be careful and do your reserach. Remember how ephedra, a stimulant that encourage weight loss, has led to a number of high-profile deaths in athletes that overused it.

GREEN TEA

Can green tea really help you lose weight? In a word: yes. Green tea has been a medicinal beverage in Asia for almost 4,000 years. The tea leaf itself has an abundance of vitamins, minerals and antioxidants. The extract is a highly concentrated part of the camellia sinensis leaf, a perennial evergreen shrub.

Green tea increases fat oxidation and thermogenesis without an increase in your heart rate. It also acts as a diuretic, safely removing excess water from the body that can lead to a bloated look. It also lets your body selectively burn fat while sparing lean mass.

There are many brands of green tea. There are also varying amounts of green tea in "serving sizes" and some teas claim they have "lots of vitamins added." You don't need more vitamins; you need more green tea added to get the job done. Green tea comes in bags, loose tea and capsules. Capsules are the best as they can contain more green tea and they are fast and easy to take: You don't have to stop everything to brew, sit and drink to get the weight loss effect of green tea.

NUTRITION FOR OBESITY

We know obesity is basically caused by eating too much food. But some obese people may have an inadequate amount of all the essential vitamins and minerals in their bodies, which can cause difficulties in routinely burning fat. So it's important not only to worry about the number of calories you consume, but also about eating the proper foods for the balance of vitamins and minerals that can help you lose weight.

PSYLLIUM SEED HUSKS PROVIDE FIBER AND CUT DOWN HUNGER PANGS.

CHROMIUM PICOLINATE REDUCES SUGAR CRAVINGS BY STABILIZING THE METABOLISM OF SIMPLE CARBOHYDRATES.

KELP AIDS IN WIGHT LOSS THROUGH BALANCED MINERALS AND IODINE.

LECITHIN IS A FAT EMULSIFIER THAT BREAKS DOWN FAT SO IT CAN BE REMOVED FROM THE BODY.

BREAD AS A DIET AID

I'm tired of hearing people say that bread is not good for you. I love bread and have eaten it all my life at almost every meal. There are so many vitamin-rich breads that taste so good you do not even need butter. I rarely eat white bread, though.

One of the biggest mysteries to me is why people on a diet will pass on the bread or rolls, yet order food laden with calories and fat, and wolf it all down.

Bread itself is not fattening. An average slice contains 70 calories, an average roll 113 calories. Bread is filling and helps reduce the craving for higher calorie foods during the meal. A baked potato, for example, has 104 calories; with butter, add another 100 calories; and with sour cream, add yet another 150 calories. A Big Mac has 590 calories; a Double Whopper with cheese, 1,010 calories!

It's easy to see how a roll with just a little butter can replace many calories (and fat). My favorite restaurant meal is a roll, 2 appetizers, one of which I take as my main course, and then sometimes a dessert, which I often share with my tablemates. Once in a while, if I decide to have an appetizer and a main course, I will steal a bite of someone else's dessert...but I always eat my bread. The texture, flavor and taste of bread should be savored, so eat slowly.

For family dinner dieting, buy the best enriched rolls or bread. Choose your bread as carefully as you would linger over a piece of meat to serve for dinner, or pick over the vegetables to get the best. Encourage your family to eat a roll. At the same time, cook and serve less meat and other high calorie foods at the table. It's healthier and you'll save money.

For lunch, have a sandwich. Choose nutritious bread. Be careful though, if you are on a strict diet. Some bread products are higher in calories: a 2-ounce muffin contains 165 calories; a 2-ounce croissant, 240 calories. Put some cold cuts in between the bread, keep the butter and mayo low, use a little mustard for added flavor and put some lettuce and tomato on it—yum. Take that, fat cells!

THE AMERICAN WAY OF DIETING

So far I have said nothing about diets to control your weight. The reason is that I don't believe in them. Something is very wrong with the way Americans try to control their weight. We tend to overeat, pick the newest popular diet to lose the weight, then overeat and diet again.

Which diet-of-the-month might you be currently counting on to bring your weight into line with your goals? There are a lot out there: Atkins, Low Carbohydrate, South Beach, Beverly Hills, Pritikin, Cabbage Soup, Jenny Craig, Fit for Life, Glycemic Index, Nutrisystem, Scarsdale, Slim-Fast, Sugar Busters, Suzanne Somers, Weight Watchers, The Zone, Revival Soy, Subway—and I could list dozens more. There is no lack of choices, and there will be a new one being promoted tomorrow and next week! Yet people keep getting fatter.

Whether you choose one of the formal diets above or pop a pill, you lose weight only if you expend more calories than you ingest. You will not be able to exercise enough to counteract overeating. We are not chopping wood, washing our laundry by hand or hunting for our food out in the wild these days. You must learn to see the plate of food sitting in front of you as a possible enemy...one that can help kill you.

I believe the exercise portion of any diet program is as important as the diet itself. At the same time, proper nutrition from vitamins, minerals and trace minerals keeps your cells in tune, which in turn helps you maintain your weight. The right kind of acid/alkaline ratio allows your body to release stored fat. Alkalizing your body prepares it for weight loss and weight maintenance. A body in a high acid state will hold onto the stores of fat, making it difficult to lose weight.

So dieting is not just a matter of eating less to lose weight. It is a combination of good nutrition, exercise, and perhaps even some lifestyle changes.

My Personal "No Diet" Diet

Remember the publisher who wanted me to write a diet book, but I declined because it would only have 3 words? Well, today, I would expand that to 2 sentences: "Keep your mouth shut! Eat healthy, balanced meals, just eat less."

Well, that has been my diet for 50 years and, during that whole time, my weight has fluctuated only by a pound or 2. I'll tell you why it works.

- It's simple—I have nothing to memorize and I do not deprive myself of the foods I love. I just eat smaller portions.

- It does not require any alteration of my lifestyle. There is no need for a lot of time and energy to do advance planning or special shopping, special cooking or setting up a diet "system."

- I eat normal food and all foods, including what many diets declare off-limits. For example, most diets eliminate oil-containing foods that are essential for healthy hair, skin and nails.

- I do not eat "fat free" foods or substitutes for butter and sugar. To me they taste terrible. Just because an item says it's fat free doesn't mean you can eat more of it, as some people do. I use sugar in moderation—it builds energy, which helps burn calories.

That's it. Keep your mouth shut! Eat healthy, balanced meals, just eat less.

What do I mean by eat less? Consume less than you have been eating before. Not less than someone else. A person who does more physical labor most likely needs a higher food intake than someone sitting behind a desk all day. So you must start with the amount of food you were eating before you took on this no-diet diet. If you were eating 3 heaping tablespoons of mashed potatoes at a meal, cut it down to 2. This includes the gravy, too. If you eat 2 cookies after dinner, now eat one. It's so simple.

There can be no cheating here—the cells in your body tell on you and are a dead giveaway. You might be able to fool your brain, but you will not fool the results—or your friends. Feed your cells less, and you will lose the weight.

If you do eat too much at a meal, like an oversized portion or an extra food item, there's no reason to panic and feel that you've blown your whole diet—you haven't. You can adjust for it no later than the next day. That way you can have a night out in a fancy restaurant or get through a holiday season without worry.

> THERE IS NO MAGIC TO TAKING THE WEIGHT OFF. YOU MUST EAT LESS. IF THAT DOESN'T WORK, THEN YOU MUST EAT EVEN LESS!

But don't gauge your portions at home by the ones served in restaurants. For example, if you wanted to treat yourself to an occasional steak at a fine steak house, many of them don't offer less than a 16-ounce New York strip or a 12-ounce filet mignon. Take half of it home, or do as I do—share it with your husband or other dining partners.

As a side note, keep in mind that Americans just eat too much food in general. For instance, the average American eats about 275 pounds of meat per year; whereas the average Chinese eats only approximately 154 pounds of meat per year.

Remember, it will get easier as you go along. The beginning of any change is always the most difficult. The more weight you lose, the easier it will be to lose more. And you'll be getting more and more energy, because there will be less of you to carry around. And this means that this newfound energy can be put right to work to burn up even more calories! One very encouraging note: As your stomach shrinks, the less food you will be able to—or want to—eat.

10 TIPS FOR LOSING WEIGHT!

Besides eating less of the right foods and exercising, these tips will help you speed up the weight loss process. If you make them part of your lifestyle, they'll help you keep the weight off and make dieting easier for a lifetime.

1. Put your fork down after each bite and take the time to enjoy the flavor and sensation of the food. Rushing even a snack doesn't give your brain enough time to recognize when your stomach is full.

2. Chew thoroughly and s-l-o-w-l-y. This has the same effect as No. 1.

3. Slice your food on your plate into small pieces, eating one piece before slicing another. Put your knife and fork down while chewing and swallowing. Don't pick them up again until you're completely finished with one piece and ready to slice the next. This will really slow you down.

4. Ignore experts who say you need a big breakfast when on a diet. The more you eat, the more you want to eat. Satisfy morning hunger with a small breakfast. Then, if necessary, have a tiny snack at mid-morning. It's better to eat 5 very small meals a day than 3 big ones.

5. Don't give up your favorite food. You won't make it for long depriving yourself that way, so why try? Just eat a lot less of it and don't feel guilty. I love certain candy, so I take out 1 or 2 pieces, close the bag and put it away. If the bag isn't right there, I don't suffer from the "just-one-more" syndrome.

6. Be aware that sight and sound can trigger the brain's hunger reflex. When this happens, you can train yourself to switch thoughts or change activities to occupy your mind with something else. Sometimes just drinking a glass of water or juice will kill the desire for more food.

7. Use a luncheon plate at all meals rather than a larger dinner plate. Remember, the less you eat, the less you will want to eat because your stomach will shrink and will not want or need as much anymore.

8. Leave the dinner table hungry, and in 20 minutes you won't be hungry anymore. It takes the brain that long to register food entering your digestive system and still hunger impulses. Another method is to stretch your meals out. Take half the normal portion, and eat it slowly over the course of 20 minutes. You'll feel full! Have you ever been interrupted in the middle of a meal, then, on returning to the table, realized that you didn't feel like eating anymore? It's the same principal at work.

9. Make your snacks healthy ones. My favorite is fruit yogurt, which I keep on hand in a variety of flavors. It sure beats reaching for the potato chips. It's tastier, healthier and fills me up.

10. Don't eat standing up. Make it a rule. If you have to sit down to eat, you'll do it more slowly and maybe less often.

What to do about Cellulite?

I'm frequently asked about cellulite. That's only natural, since it is estimated that 85% of women develop it. Men are less likely to have it, because they have thicker skin, which does a better job hiding the fat beneath it. It seems to be a natural by-product of aging. There must be millions of dollars spent every year on "cellulite problems."

Simply put, cellulite is fat, the same as any other fat on your body. The term (from Latin *cellula,* "little cell") refers to the dimpled appearance of the skin seen in areas of the hips, thighs and buttocks, but it actually is an increased ratio of fat cells to lean body mass, formed by a system-wide failure to eliminate fibrous proteins that accumulate between the cells. It may become more prevalent at times because of a hormonal surge, for example, during pregnancy.

There are plenty of cellulite treatments. They are listed below, but I will tell you in advance that some are expensive and none are permanent, except perhaps one that has not yet been proven safe. Some don't work at all. You must exercise caution, since some of the unproven treatments could be potentially dangerous.

Exercise and Diet

Exercising, eating a healthy diet, and maintaining a normal weight may work as a cellulite treatment for some people. Experts suggest following a whole-foods diet with fewer complex carbohydrates and sugars than usually recommended, drinking large amounts of filtered water, decreasing fats to below 20% of the total diet, and avoiding animal fats and processed fats as much as possible. Whole foods include vegetables, fruits, whole grains, nuts, and legumes.

Self-massage of the affected area regularly might help and can be done easily at home. Let gravity assist by propping your legs up against a wall or over a chair and then massaging, very lightly, the crease formed by the legs and the abdomen in order to open the channels for the elimination of the fibrous proteins loosened by the exercise and massage.

But while exercise and diet can help, they won't solve the problem completely.

CREAMS

There are many creams on the market touted as cellulite treatments. Most are available over the counter and only a few require prescriptions. Most of them contain some fancy sounding ingredient, like prehistoric mud or the pollen of the rarest of Alpine weeds, etc.

Doctors say these creams may work for some people. Any results, however, are temporary, and the best ones are those containing theophylline or caffeine, which some studies have shown cause fat cells to dissolve.

A combination of such creams with a self-massage of the affected areas may work best. The cream will help dissolve the cellulite and release the surrounding proteins, while the massage increases circulation, aiding the process of elimination.

ENDERMOLOGIE

One of the best known cellulite treatments is endermologie, a deep-massage therapy that uses a device that suctions the skin with a vacuum and kneads it with a set of rollers. The deep tissue massage can break up some of the fibrous bands, help circulation, and improve the appearance of the skin. While it works for some women, the effects don't last. Regular maintenance—usually weekly sessions—is needed to keep up appearances. Individual treatments on average cost more than $100. Some people will get no results.

MESOTHERAPY

Mesotherapy involves a series of injections into small pockets of cellulite with a solution of homeopathic medications and supplements that supposedly break down fat and "flush" it away. Widely accepted in Europe, it has yet to be studied scientifically in the U.S., but there's a good deal of skepticism. A lot of injections heighten the risk of side effects and problems. The treatment is very expensive, costing perhaps 5 times as much as endermologie.

HERBAL MEDICINES

No combination of herbs or vitamins is known to have any effect on cellulite whatsoever, except perhaps as an aid to diet and weight.

Liposuction

Liposuction doesn't work for cellulite either. Liposuction can really only get at fat deposits deep beneath the skin. Cellulite is generally too close to the surface for liposuction to help.

Because the fibrous bands are what give cellulite its appearance, getting rid of fat alone won't do much.

A Novel Attack

An Italian clothing company released the first line of anti-cellulite pants. As you walk around town, the friction between your body and the jeans releases an anti-cellulite cream. Price: $139. The world's dermatologists are unconvinced. So am I.

The Latest

A number of cellulite treatment devices have been developed that combine deep tissue massage with other features, such as light and radio frequency therapy. Such a system received FDA approval a couple years ago, but success has been mixed at best, from less than 30% to 50%, depending on the patient and the degree of the condition. One clinician reported a better than 50% success rate when limiting patients to those who are non-smokers, not diabetic, not overweight, or without thick skin—how many women who have cellulite are left? To achieve results they had to agree to 2 sessions a week for 4 to 5 weeks. Results are not permanent and the cost can range between $1,500 to $3,000.

My Opinion

Since you can't get rid of cellulite permanently, maybe a change of attitude might be best. The next time you're looking over your shoulder, staring unhappily at the reflection of your backside in your bedroom mirror, remember this: If 85% of the women of the world have cellulite, so, too, do 85% of the most beautiful among them, including movie stars and other celebrities. Maybe you should not be so hard on yourself!!

AFTERTHOUGHTS

I'm tired of all the chatter about weight loss: "I can't lose weight no matter how hard I try." "I eat like a bird and still can't lose weight." "I lost 10 pounds, but gained back 12." "It's hard, so hard." It's as if there's an I-can't-lose-weight society that people buy into and support each other over remaining overweight. Membership in that club will kill you.

I don't mean to sound harsh. I just want to get you thinking in another direction. There is no magic to taking the weight off. You must eat less. If that doesn't work, then you must eat even less! Of course this puts the responsibility on you—and that is where it belongs. No one else can do it for you.

I have friends of all sizes and shapes. I love them all and they'll always be part of my life, but I give them the same advice I'm giving you: Deprive yourself now of a little food, or be deprived later of your health and well-being.

CHAPTER 9

EXERCISE

"Excuse" is our biggest enemy.

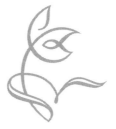

I don't know many people who like to exercise…I know I don't. What keeps me going is that, if I'm going to stay looking and feeling young for as long as possible—and I certainly intend to—I cannot give up my flexibility.

Some people force themselves to exercise to lose weight, but that will not keep you motivated in the long run, and it is only half the battle. Remember that you also must eat less and consume the proper foods in order to lose weight

If you are into tennis, swimming, biking or any other aerobic sport, that certainly counts. You do not have to be at the gym every day "sweating it out" to have a healthy body—but, if you like it, so much the better. In general, almost any exercise that you stick with will be beneficial.

Living without some form of exercise will lead to poor health, and probably sooner than you think. A physical breakdown may be repaired by a doctor, perhaps through the use of medications—perhaps with side effects—but that's not the answer. If you want to be preventative, exercise regularly and watch your diet. Exercising is one of the best anti-aging pastimes you can engage in.

DANGERS OF JOGGING, RUNNING AND JUMPING

If you or a loved one are a serious jogger or runner, consider stopping being one. The force of impact with the ground puts between 3 and 5 times your body weight on your feet and ankles, and the long-range effects on your body can create problems that can never be undone

I never ran or jogged, but I was an excellent rope jumper. That was my form of exercise. I even did it on live TV once in a contest with the host. He was a jogger and claimed he was in better shape than me because of it. Well, he was exhausted after 10 or so jumps and completely out of breath. I went on until the host told me he was running out of time!

However, jumping rope, like running and jogging, is not a safe way to exercise. Oh, perhaps teenagers and people in their early 20s can get away with it for a while, but the effects of repetitive pounding on your feet, knees, bones, ligaments, tendons, joints and lower back and hips will develop problems that can stay with you for life.

Some years ago, my doctor told me that bouncing/jumping up and down also can cause a woman's organs to drop down. In time, they could press against my bladder and cause incontinence, a problem many women experience as they grow older. My doctor was emphatic that I should stop jumping rope immediately—I did—and it paid off. At age 75 I have not had any problems! If you or a loved one are running or jogging—or jumping rope—stop. The payoff for you or them is worth it.

THE BEST ALTERNATIVE: WALKING

Walk fast—even very fast—outdoors or on a treadmill.

Walking is a workout with no disadvantages. Almost anyone can do it, with little chance of injury. You can walk practically anywhere, either alone or with a friend or family member, and it requires no special equipment unless you prefer a treadmill.

Walking can also be a great aerobic workout for the body's cardiovascular system, and it reduces body fat. Walking tones and firms the hips and thighs. It develops the calf and shin muscles better than running, toning the entire length of the muscles and helping them stay lean.

As with all forms of exercise, correct form will enhance the effectiveness of the workout. Good posture allows you to move quickly. Stand erect to protect the lower back and improve your abdominal strength. The foot action is a heel strike followed by rolling onto the ball of the foot and pushing off the toes.

Swing the arms from the shoulder and shorten their angle to 90 degrees in order to move faster. The faster pace may feel difficult to hold at first; your shins may fatigue. Make a goal of walking at least 3 times a week minimum for overall good health.

If you were a serious jogger or runner, you might try the following.

- The first week start out with 1 or 2 miles. If you have not exercised for some time, don't overdo the speed for the first week. Build up to it. Toward the end slow down and stroll for the last 5 minutes. Do not stop abruptly.

- Gradually increase the distance each day and walk faster until you're walking about 3 miles at a steady brisk pace.

Keep up the regimen. You'll be amazed at how good you'll feel in a short time.

You may find it difficult to walk outdoors in inclement weather, freezing cold or blazing heat. On days like that, try driving to an enclosed shopping mall. If you arrive there early before the stores open, you'll find the mall empty, and you can speed walk under cover in heated or air conditioned space, and do some window shopping at the same time. It is fun with a friend or a group, and you'll find you won't be alone, since mall walking has become popular around the country. The stores like it, too, because you might see something that you will want to buy later.

Want Your Waistline Back?

Are you losing weight but not slimming your waistline? I was always amazed as a young girl to watch my mother doing some exercises that she said trimmed her waistline. I wrote about it in my book, *How To Renovate Yourself From Head To Toe*, more than 20 years ago and had forgotten about it until someone asked me how to get a smaller waistline. My mother's simple routine is still valid today, so let me share it with you.

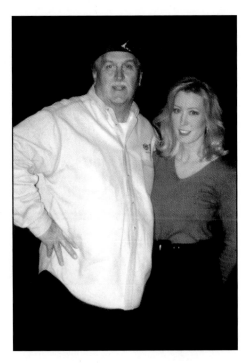

OLEDA, AGE 66,
AND HER BROTHER,
HARRY, 63

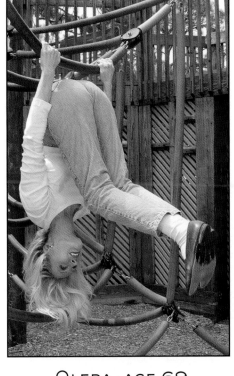

OLEDA, AGE 69

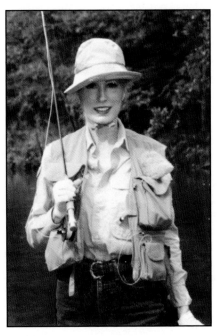

ON A FISHING TRIP,
AGE 63

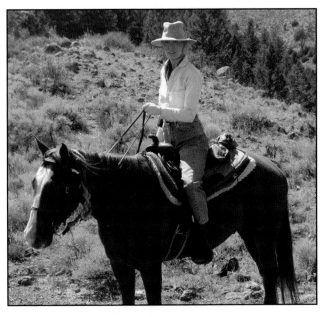

HORSEBACK RIDING, AGE 74

OLEDA AGE 26-75

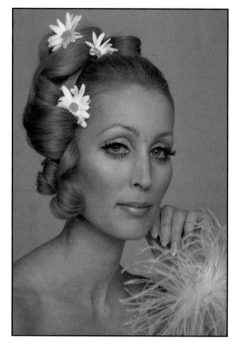

26

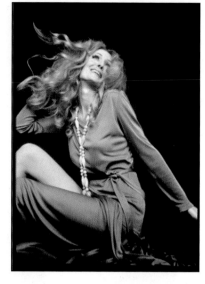

30

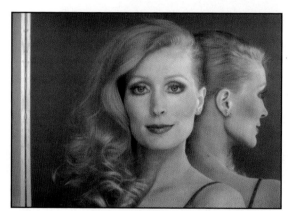

45

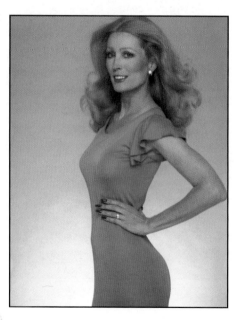

48

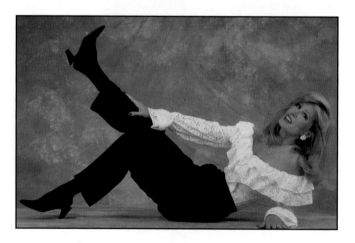

59

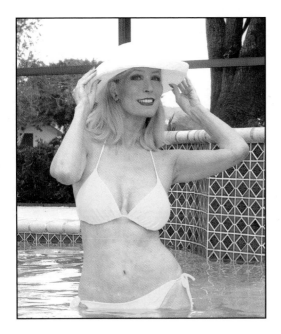

69

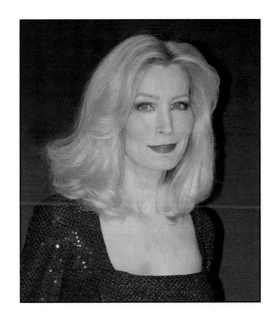

69

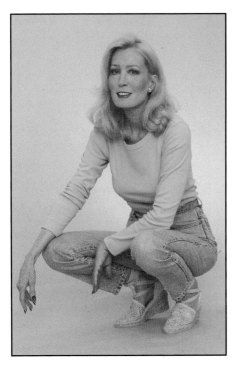

71

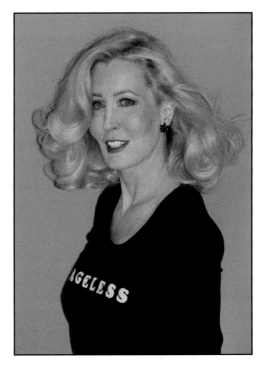

75

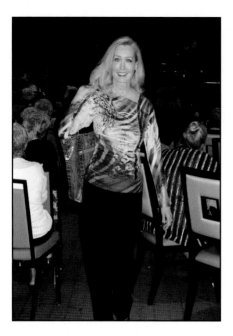

MODELING AT A CHARITY
FASHION SHOW,
AGE 75

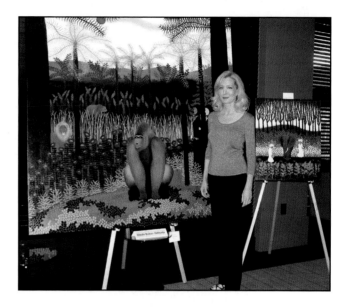

WITH SOME OF HER
PAINTINGS, AGE 74

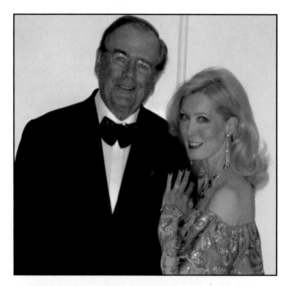

OLEDA AND HER HUSBAND,
RICHARD, BOTH AT 71

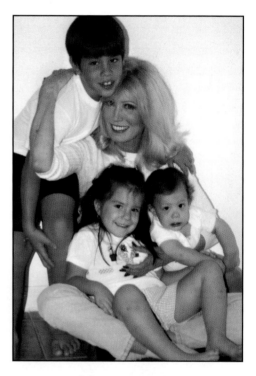

NANA, 66,
WITH GRANDCHILDREN
DAVID, ALISON AND SEAN

1. Standing with your feet about 18 inches apart, hold arms straight out, parallel to the floor. Keeping your feet planted, twist from the waist in any direction, swinging your arms as far back as they will go. Hold for one second, press backward another inch and return to starting position. Stop one second and repeat in the opposite direction. Do this 10 times for each side.

2. Assuming the same position as in step 1, stretch one arm straight down toward the floor (right arm trying to reach right foot) and the other toward the ceiling as far as you can. Stop 1 second, press another inch and return to starting position. Stop 1 second, repeat on the other side of your body. Do 10 repetitions.

3. Still standing with your feet about 18 inches apart, raise your arms straight up over your head as far as they will go. Bend both hands at the wrists until palms are facing the ceiling. Then, slowly s-t-r-e-t-c-h up as far as you can, keeping your feet firmly planted. Hold this position for 5 seconds, stretch up 1 more inch, then relax and assume the starting position. Do this 10 times.

4. Sit with your ankles crossed, leaning on your left hand, elbow slightly bent. Raise your right arm straight up over your head with palm facing upward and force it as far as you can toward your left side, feeling the stretch in your right waist. Hold for 5 seconds. Repeat on the other side of your body. Do this 6 times on each side.

Do this routine every day for a month or 2, then 3 or 4 times a week. You'll see the difference!

7 Steps to Firm Flabby Arms

Flabby upper arms are caused by extra fat and loose skin. It's not too easy to get rid of, but it can be done.

Being overweight can contribute to flabby arms, so if you're flabby elsewhere, your arms could likely be the same way. You will need to diet every day, taking in fewer calories than you burn. You may lose weight elsewhere before you see much of an effect on your arms. Whether you're overweight or not, exercising the triceps a minimum of 3 times a week should be your main effort in getting rid of flabby arms.

Follow this regimen.

1. Sit on the front edge of a chair. Your feet should be flat on the floor, spaced apart so that they are even with your shoulders.

2. Hold a weight in one hand. A small, 5-pound one will do (it's not so much the weight that counts, but doing the repetitions). Raise your left arm all the way up, so that it's pointing toward the ceiling, palm facing in. You can support your left arm by holding it just below the elbow with your right hand.

3. Slowly bend your arm so that the weight in your hand now rests behind your shoulder. Take 3 seconds to straighten your arm so that it's pointing toward the ceiling again. Hold the position for 1 second.

4. Take 3 seconds to lower the weight back to your shoulder by bending your elbow. Keep supporting your arm with your other hand throughout the exercise.

5. Pause, and then repeat the bending and straightening until you have done the exercise 8 to 15 times.

6. Change hands and repeat 8 to 15 times with your other arm.

7. Rest; then do another 2 sets of 8 to 15 repetitions on each side.

The number of repetitions depends on your strength level. Start slowly at 8, and then build up to 15 according to your comfort level. You'll be surprised at how quickly that happens. If you can, then go to 20; the idea is to fatigue the triceps. It might take a while, but depending on how flabby your arms are, you should begin to see results in about 4 weeks.

For women who have lost a lot of weight and suffered an abnormal amount of flabbiness under their upper arms as a result, exercising the triceps in this fashion will not work. They might consider investigating alternative methods.

- Thermage, a skin-tightening procedure that uses radio frequency.

- Liposuction and surgery after liposuction to remove excess skin (although there will be scarring).

FOR A FLEXIBLE BACK

If your back is tight, the rest of your body suffers with it. A painful back can cause you to stoop, making you look and feel older. It might even require medication that could have been avoided. Stretching can help you avoid back pain, and can keep your body more agile throughout your life.

I do the following exercises 2 or 3 times a week, skipping a week here and there. Don't worry if you can't go as far as I do in these photos. You can build up to it sooner than you think.

SET ONE

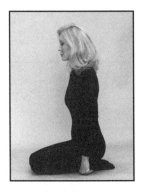

1. Sit on legs.

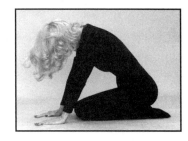

2. Bend forward putting hands flat on floor.

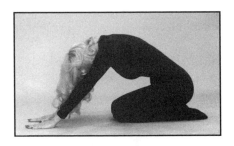

3. Scoot hands forward and stretch out keeping hands flat on floor.

4. Bend over stretching out as far as you can, keeping hands and elbows on floor. You will feel your lower back stretching. Hold for a few seconds. Do 5 repetitions.

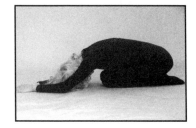

SET TWO

1. Lie on your back—knees up.

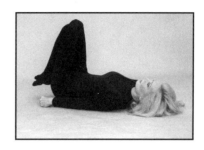

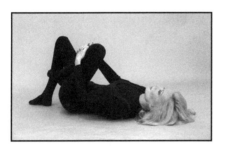

2. Pull knees up toward your chest one leg at a time.

3. Gently, press knee as far as you can toward your chest...hold for a few seconds. Do one leg at a time, and then do both legs at the same time. Do 5 repetitions of each.

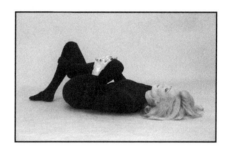

SET THREE

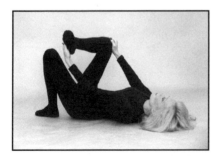

Lift one leg, pull foot toward you with one hand while gently pushing the bent knee outward with the other. Hold for a few seconds. Do 5 repetitions.

OTHER GOOD STRETCHING POSITIONS

(When you are ready)

Here is another stretching exercise I do, when your body can easily accommodate the first 3 exercises I've described. Be sure, though, you are somewhat limber already and have a friend or trainer watching or guiding you. Do not force it.

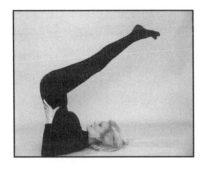

1. Raise your bottom up as shown, supported by your hands.

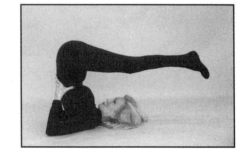

2. Extend your legs back and straight as far as possible.

3. Bend knees downward still supporting yourself at the waist.

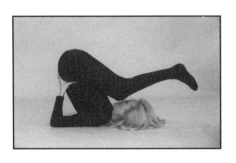

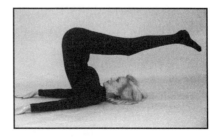

4. Carefully drop your arms to the floor palms down.

5. Hold for a count of 5 and then very slowly lower your bottom back to the floor. Relax.

Simple Stretching and Weight Training Exercises

For strength building and flexibility exercises, having a gym is nice, but you can do them at home, too. The key to any strength building routine is resistance and repetition.

You will need 2 dumbbells. Start with 3- to 5-pound weights, or ones you can lift comfortably 8 to 12 times. Doing 1 set is beneficial, but work up to 3 sets. Lifting the weights should not be effortless. When it becomes too easy, move up to heavier weights; but don't overdo it. If you can't repeat an exercise 8 times, the weight is too heavy. The key is to fatigue your muscles, and this is done best through repetition. Three 20-minute sessions a week will do the job. Avoid doing it on consecutive days, though.

If you want to speed up the effectiveness of the exercises, eat a combination of carbs and protein about 2 hours before you exercise and immediately after. This can increase the benefit by up to 25%. Begin with the stretching instruction below for each part of the body, and then proceed to the weight training.

Upper Body Stretches

Hand Press

- Sit on a chair with your feet flat on the floor. Press your palms together in front of your chest so your elbows are pointed out to the sides.

- Keeping your hands pressed together, drop them down and toward your stomach until you feel a stretch in your wrists and forearms. Hold for 20 seconds. Do 8 to 12 repetitions.

Sit and Reach

- Sit tall in a chair with your feet flat on the floor. Place your right hand on your left upper arm above the elbow.

- Twist to the right and grasp the back of the chair seat with your left hand, bringing your chin over your right shoulder as you turn. Hold for 15 seconds and switch sides. Do 8 to 12 repetitions.

SLUMP DOWN

- Sit on the edge of a chair with your knees spread slightly and your feet directly below your knees.

- Slump your body forward over your legs so your chest rests on or above your knees and your arms hang down. Wrap your arms under your knees and press your back up toward the ceiling while keeping your chest on the knees. Hold this position for 20 to 30 seconds. Do 8 to 12 repetitions.

UPPER BODY EXERCISE

CHEST AND UPPER ARMS

- Stand holding dumbbells in each hand and lift arms straight out to the sides. Now bend your arms to 90-degree angles keeping your hands about head level. Palms of hands should face front holding the dumbbells.

- While squeezing your chest muscles, move your elbows slowly toward each other until they're about shoulder width apart in front of you. Return to the starting position. Do 8 to 12 repetitions.

PECTORAL MUSCLE SQUEEZE

- Holding a dumbbell in your right hand, stand with your left leg one large step in front of your right, with your back heel lifted off the floor. Rest your left hand on your left thigh for balance and lean forward slightly. Hold your right arm across your chest so your palm faces toward your back.

- Keeping your elbow bent, move it out to the side and up until your upper arm is parallel with the floor (even with your shoulder). Pause, then return to the starting position. After doing 8 to 12 repetitions change sides and repeat the exercise with the other arm.

CURLS

- Sit on an armless chair with your feet flat on the floor. Hold a dumbbell in each hand with your arms extended down at your sides, palms facing your thighs.

- Keeping your upper body stable, bend your elbows and curl the weights up toward your shoulders.

- Immediately rotate your wrists so your palms are facing away from you and push the weights overhead.

- Pause, then reverse the move, lowering the weights to your shoulders, rotating your palms in toward your body. Lower the weights back down to your sides. Do 8 to 12 repetitions.

Triceps

- Hold a dumbbell in your left hand. Stand beside a chair and place your right knee and hand on the seat so you're bent over with your chest parallel to the floor. Hold your left elbow at your side so your arm is bent at a 90-degree angle and your forearm is perpendicular to the floor.

- Extend your elbow backwards until your forearm is parallel to the floor. Pause 5 seconds, then lower to the starting position. Complete 8 to12 repetitions, and then switch sides.

Lower Body Stretch

Lunges

- Stand with your feet together with your right hand on a wall for support.

- Take a giant step back with your right leg, keeping the heel off the floor.

- Gently bend your left leg and drop your hips toward the floor, pressing your pelvis forward until you feel a gentle stretch down the front of your right hip and leg. Hold for 15 to 20 seconds and switch sides. Do 8 to 12 repetitions.

Calf Stretch

- Stand at arm's length from a wall and place your palms flat against it. Extend your left leg behind you about 24 to 36 inches and press your left heel to the floor. Your right knee will bend naturally as you extend the other leg.

- Keeping both heels flat against the floor, press against the wall until you feel a nice stretch in your calf. Hold for 15 seconds, and then repeat with the other leg. Do 8 to 12 repetitions.

THIGH STRETCH

- Sit on the floor with your back straight, your knees bent and the soles of your feet touching so your knees fall out to the sides.

- Grasp your ankles with your hands. Keeping your back straight, gently bend forward from the hips as you press your knees down toward the floor as far as comfortably possible. Hold for 20 to 30 seconds. Do 8 to 12 repetitions.

- Standing upright, place your left heel about 12 inches in front of you, point your toes up and lean forward. Place your hands on your right thigh for support.

HAMSTRING STRETCH

- Bend your right knee and gently bend forward from the hips, pressing your weight back until you feel a stretch in the back of your left leg. Hold for 15 seconds, and then switch legs. Do 8 to 12 repetitions on each side.

LOWER BODY EXERCISE

POWER PULL

- Stand with your feet hip-width apart, holding a light dumbbell in your left hand. Squat until your legs are bent at about 45 degrees and place your right hand on your right thigh for support. Reach across your body with your left arm, holding the dumbbell in front of your right knee.

- In one smooth motion, pull your arm back across your body (as though starting a motor with a pull cord) and stand up slightly, though not fully. Squat back down and repeat 5 times. Then switch sides.

LEG LIFT

- Sit on the floor with your legs extended in front of you, your back straight and your feet flexed. Place your hands on your lap or on the floor behind you for support.

- Keeping your foot flexed, tighten your left thigh and slowly raise your left heel off the floor.

- Pause, and then slowly return to the starting position. Complete 8 to 12 repetitions, and then switch legs.

SLIDING SQUATS

- Stand with your back against a wall with your legs straight and your feet about 24 inches from the wall and slightly apart. Raise your arms straight out in front of you and slide down the wall until your thighs are nearly parallel to the floor.

- Hold for 3 to 5 seconds. Slide back up to the starting position, lowering your arms as you stand. Do 5 repetitions.

CALF BUILDER

- Stand on the bottom step of a flight of stairs. Lightly grasp the banister, or place your hand on a wall for support. Bend your right leg and place the toes of your left foot on the edge of the step.

- Let your left heel drop as far as comfortably possible. Press into the ball of your left foot and raise yourself onto your toes. Pause, and then return to the starting position. Complete 8 to 12 repetitions, and then switch legs.

AFTERTHOUGHTS

Research has shown that older women—70-plus—can do successful strength training.[13] In fact, older muscles are quite responsive; the real problem is low expectations. The benefits of building and preserving muscle are manifold, including preventing serious falls, building a better immune system and a faster metabolism. So go ahead! Pump up! Three 20-minute sessions a week (preferably not on consecutive days) will do the job.

CHAPTER 10

MENTAL ATTITUDE

The mind is your most powerful weapon against aging.

Years ago it was thought that when we were born we had all the brain cells we were ever going to have. However, toward the end of the 20th century, researchers demonstrated that people can grow new brain cells and new neurons as adults, even in old age.[14]

The truth is that memory, as well as the rate at which we process information, does start to decline in our 40s. But the drop-off is less than most of us make of it. Experts attribute cognitive decline during those years to factors unrelated to anything physical; instead it's the kids, work, bills, chores, e-mail, etc., all competing for time in our heads, making it more difficult to devote the attention required to learn something new or recall something already learned. So, if you've already reached your 40s, don't worry—but, as you grow older, pay attention.

To keep your brain young you need to give it lots of varied stimulation and challenges. Like a muscle, it needs to be exercised, to "strain the brain," so to speak. Repeating the same mental functions over and over, such as playing cards or watching television, doesn't help slow cognitive deterioration. Mental stimulation is as important for your brain as physical exercise is for your body.

When my grandmother passed away at age 95, her mind was still sharp as a tack. She stayed busy all her life with church matters. In her late 80s she took the "old people" to the doctor and to the store, and brought them food when they were sick. She also helped paint the outside of her daughter's house. Until she was 94, she walked a couple of miles most days. When she died she had a fruit and vegetable garden, a flower garden and was going to church 3 times a week.

For me there is nothing I won't try—well, maybe there's one: singing, which makes my friends happy! I had no idea I could develop and run a business. When I stumbled onto an opportunity at age 38, I ran with it. Nearly 40 years later, I'm still CEO of Oleda and Company, Inc, and I love the challenges that come with that job.

I always had a desire to put my feelings on canvas but had no idea if I could paint, so I picked up a paint brush when I was almost 40 and gave it a try. Since then I've had 2 museum exhibitions and several gallery shows, and sold lots of paintings (even though I hate to let them go).

I live by the slogan, "You have to be in it to win it." How can you know that you can't do something if you don't try?

How To Save Your Brain... Or Reinvent It!

You might think the most important deterrent to brain cell deterioration is engaging in mind-bending games or doing the daily crossword puzzle. Taxing the brain and learning new skills are excellent activities, but they usually don't get your heart rate up and pump blood to your brain cells.

Perhaps the most striking brain research discovery of the last decade is that exercise can forestall mental decline.[15] It may even restore memory. Animal studies have shown that aerobic exercise increases capillary development in the brain, increasing blood supply, which carries more oxygen to the brain.

But it doesn't have to be formal exercise at the gym. You can play tennis a couple times a week, ride a bike, or walk a mile each day. If you want to get really serious about it, though, a combined program of aerobics and weight training (anaerobic exercise) will produce the best results.

Fit people have sharper brains; and people who are out of shape but then get into shape sharpen their brains as well as their bodies.

NUTRITION FOR A HEALTHY BRAIN

To function properly the brain needs glucose, sodium, potassium, unsaturated fatty acids, amino acids (protein), vitamins, minerals and at least 400 calories a day.

We've all heard about antioxidants as cancer fighters. Eating foods that contain these substances, which neutralize harmful free radicals, are especially good for your brain, too. Free radicals break down the neurons in your brain, so the many colorful fruits and vegetables that are packed with antioxidants are good for you in more ways than one.

Too much alcohol has been linked to brain atrophy, because it causes direct injury to the cells. The good news is that these cells can be rebuilt when people eliminate alcohol from the diet.

Scientists have shown that certain nutrients are essential for human brain function. Serious deficiencies in vitamin B12 and iron, for example, can lead to impaired cognition due to neurological or nerve fiber complications. Paying careful attention to diet helps protect the brain from developing problems with nerve cell signals that are involved in memory and cognition.

Food with high oxygen radical absorbance capacity (ORAC) scores are thought to help improve cognition. The score includes all the antioxidants in foods and indentifies which are the important ones. An ORAC score of around 5,000 units per day can have a significant effect on blood and tissue antioxidant levels.

THE FOLLOWING FRUITS HAVE THE HIGHEST ORAC SCORES (NUMBERS ARE BASED ON 1/2 CUP OF EACH):

PRUNES: 7,290

BLUEBERRIES: 6,500

BLACK PLUMS: 4,500

BLACKBERRIES: 3,800

Other fruits and vegetables have good ORAC scores as well, but soomewhat less punch. Some food producers place ORAC scores on their products, so you can look for them as you shop.

There is promising evidence that using ginkgo biloba as a dietary supplement enhances memory. It doesn't have any harmful side effects, but it should be used with caution by those on anticoagulant therapy, or about to undergo some surgical or dental procedures.

Drink plenty of water, too. Your brain is about 80% liquid and needs to be well hydrated to function well.

BENEFITS OF A POSITIVE ATTITUDE

Both chronic and traumatic stress can actually damage your brain cells and disturb cognitive processes such as learning and memory. This is particularly true in a part of the brain called the hippocampus, a structure shaped like a sea horse whose main functions are the consolidation of new memories, spatial orientation, navigation and motivation. A relaxed, positive attitude is one of the best countermeasures.

Try to train yourself to react calmly to stressful situations. Keeping your responses as low key as possible and reacting in a firm, unexcited way will help you cope better with most situations. As CEO of my company, when a serious event occurs, I focus on the business aspect of it, not the personalities involved. This keeps my emotional stress under control and gets me to the core of the problem faster.

RELAXATION

While challenging your brain is very important, so too is "down time"—making room in your life for relaxation. It's important to stop, take deep breaths and learn to relax. I love to paint. I "step into my painting" and get lost. I also like to take a 15-minute nap during the day.

SLEEP

Do you keep a notepad and pencil on your bed stand? I don't know how many times I wake up in the morning and a bright answer pops up to a problem I was laboring over the day before. Researchers have studied the conditions under which people come up with creative solutions and found that a good night's rest doubled participants' chances of finding answers to problems.[16] The sleeping brain seems to be capable of synthesizing vast amounts of complex information.

The next time you're struggling with a problem, whether it's a complicated mathematical equation or choosing the right car for your family, it really pays to "sleep on it."

KEEPING A POSITIVE ATTITUDE

Focus on the glass being half full. If a friend disappoints you, for example, remember the times that person supported you in the past. Use that memory in dealing with the current emptiness.

Some people have a more difficult time than others in keeping a healthy, positive attitude. If you're one of them, you might only need to work a little harder to see the bright side of things. But if it's a deeper problem, you should seek professional help.

DEPRESSION

It's possible for a person to have a genetic predisposition to depression because of an imbalance of neurotransmitters, or chemicals that help send messages between nerve cells in the brain. Some of them regulate mood, and if they run low, a person can become anxious, stressed and depressed. Indeed, stress itself can magnify this imbalance, making depression more intense.

It is not unusual for such people to be affected by depression without having suffered a traumatic trigger event in their lives. If you're feeling depressed, regardless of cause—stress, genetic disposition, psychological trauma—do not hesitate to consult a doctor for help. There are medications available that will restore a proper balance in your neurotransmitters.

HOLDING A GRUDGE

Holding a grudge or harboring resentment causes brain stagnation and depletes energy. It creates emotional stress, raises your blood pressure, ages your face with frowning expressions and can affect your physical and mental well-being.

Learn to forgive, and you will free yourself of damaging negativism that robs you of vitality and beauty. Forgiving doesn't mean excusing, but understanding human frailty and seeking a higher plane from which to wish the "wrongdoer" a good life despite the hurt that he or she may have caused. It might require considering the overall good in keeping family and friends together, rather than focusing only on yourself and your personal feelings. This does not necessarily mean you should resume the relationship you had before; sometimes it's best to see less of someone who brings negativity into your life.

> *To err is human, to forgive divine.*
> —Alexander Pope
>
> *Forgive all who have offended you, not for them, but for yourself.*
> —Harriet Uts Nelson
>
> *Forgiveness is a very real beauty secret.*
> —Oleda Baker

AFTERTHOUGHTS

It was 1977. My son David and I were in a taxi in New York City on our way to a luncheon to celebrate my 43rd birthday. I don't remember how it came up, but at some point David said, "Gee, Mom, you're getting old." I turned to him and replied, "Well, let's look at it this way, either I become another year older, or I'm 6 feet under."

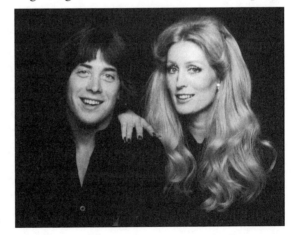

David has never repeated that statement since, although we reminisce about that incident every now and then. Now he says simply, "Love you, Mom."

I can honestly say I don't think about how many birthdays I've had. I'm too busy thinking about what I'm going to do next, having fun with the love of my life, my husband, Richard, watching my 3 grandchildren grow, and learning new things. I have no time to think about "getting old."

CHAPTER 11

REST AND RELAXATION

Don't forget your beauty sleep.

> The worst thing in the world is to try to sleep and not to.
>
> —F. Scott Fitzgerald

Judging from the mountain of mail I receive from people who cannot get a good night's sleep and wake up feeling sluggish, the problem is widespread. That's a pity because sleeplessness is a major drain on the way we look and feel. Getting proper rest at night is also essential for good health and maintaining your attractiveness. Why? Because your body eliminates dead cells and waste chemicals while you sleep and produces new cells twice as fast as when you're awake. The term "beauty sleep" is not a myth.

Smoking, drinking and exercise can affect your sleep dramatically. With some people, what they do in bed before falling asleep, such as reading, watching TV or spending time in front of the computer, affects both the quality and quantity of their sleep.

Many studies have shown that sleep deprivation adversely affects performance and alertness.[17, 18] Reducing sleep by as little as one and a half hours for just one night reduces daytime alertness by about one-third. Excessive daytime sleepiness impairs memory and the ability to think and process information, slows reflexes and increases the risk of having an accident.

American families are so much busier than they used to be. Often both parents are working and there is not enough time to do everything in a 24-hour period. As a result, many people don't get enough sleep. No wonder there is so much fatigue.

How Much Sleep Do We Really Need?

Individual needs vary, but the range lies between 6 and 1/2 hours and 9 and 1/2 hours.

How do you know if you're not getting enough sleep? You can try this simple test: Starting on a Sunday, do not drink any alcohol or caffeine, and do not smoke. For the next 6 nights, go to bed about the same time and try to get 7 to 8 hours of uninterrupted sleep. Then, on Saturday morning, sleep in. If you sleep longer than you did during the week, chances are you have a sleep deficiency and should consider getting more sleep every night.

The bottom line is that you should wake up feeling refreshed in the morning. The optimum amount of sleep allows you to function throughout the day without feeling drowsy when you sit quietly and try to focus on a project.

You can't look good and live a long life if you're not getting proper sleep. Period!

Two Common Myths

We Need Less Sleep As We Get Older

The best research available indicates that healthy older people sleep about as much as they did when they were young adults.[19] The notion that the elderly sleep less got started because of those individuals who have medical conditions that interfere with their sleep.

You Can't Make Up for Lost Sleep

You can make up for lost sleep, but only to a certain extent. After significant sleep loss, we will probably have more deep sleep for the next couple of nights, but we most likely will not sleep more than 2 to 4 hours longer than usual. This is because our wakefulness-sleep cycle depends on both our sleep need and our internal timing mechanisms.

Tired of Being Tired?

Unless you have a serious illness, you can get back the energy you once had. There is so much in life to do.

My own bout with fatigue came when I was 28 years old as a model living a fast pace in New York City. I had many assignments, so I had to keep my hair in top shape, my nails always looking good and all the other things a model has to do to keep her job! On weekends we would head out to the country for a party or stay in town for some night-clubbing. All the while, I had a home, a husband and a son to take care of. I wasn't getting enough sleep and felt exhausted much of the time.

A couple of weeks before leaving for a shoot in Italy for a major fashion magazine, I felt very tired and made an appointment with my doctor. After hearing about my life-style, he told me I was making a mistake not getting proper rest, and that if I continued at that pace, it would soon take its toll. When he discovered that I also was anemic, he gave me an injection of B-complex vitamin, recommended a B-complex supplement, and strongly suggested that I change my ways.

I heeded his advice, and by the time I arrived in Italy, I was already feeling much better—and I no longer needed extra makeup to hide a tired face. Since then I always made sure to get 7 to 8 hours of sleep every night.

Sleep Deprivation Culprits

If you're not getting enough sleep, it may be for one or more of the following reasons. The best way to deal with them is to change your lifestyle. You may not be able to do so right away, but there are some actions you can take immediately to compensate for your sluggishness.

Night Owl Habits

If you're a "night owl" or a "burner of the midnight oil" trying to squeeze more things into your busy schedule, or you're just afraid you're going to miss something by going to bed, stop! Tonight, force yourself to retire at least one hour earlier than usual, and continue going to bed at that time every night for a week.

INSOMNIA

Insomnia describes a state in which people can't fall asleep, stay asleep or sleep soundly without difficulty, no matter what time they go to bed. If you suffer from this condition and simple home remedies don't help, see your doctor. A simple lack of calcium and magnesium might cause you to wake up soon after falling asleep and prevent you from going back to sleep,

STIMULANTS

Don't take anything with caffeine in it after 4 p.m., especially coffee. Even the decaffeinated kind contains some caffeine. Also avoid soft drinks, unless it's an energy building nutritional supplement. It's best to restrict the amount of coffee and soda pop you drink during the day anyway. One or 2 cups are plenty.

CIGARETTES

If you smoke cigarettes, quit. Studies have shown that people who smoke cigarettes have more difficulty falling asleep and staying asleep because cigarettes can raise blood pressure, increase the heart rate and stimulate brain wave activity.

ALCOHOL

Excessive use of alcohol might "knock you out," but any sleep it induces will be fitful. Drink too much alcohol and you will wake up fatigued and maybe with a hangover. Make it a habit and it will destroy your beauty and shorten your life.

Women are more susceptible to the effects of alcohol than men. One drink containing one ounce of hard liquor, or one glass of wine is considered beneficial for women (men can have 2), but the danger is that, once you have one, you want more. A nice glass of wine with a meal or a cocktail beforehand is wonderful. Keep it at that.

MEDICATIONS

Some medications have side effects that can keep you awake at night and could be the cause of your fatigue. Ask your pharmacist or google them for side effects. If you're taking them for a short period, don't worry about it, but if they're regular meds, such as an anti-depressant drug, see your doctor. You must have your sleep.

Be careful about sleeping pills, though. These medications should not be taken for more than 4 weeks. Longer use leads to increased insomnia.

WORRY AND STRESS

People often lose sleep when they're bothered by something. The resulting worry and stress are not easy to overcome, but there are a few things you can try.

- When your head hits the pillow at night, focus your mind on a pleasant thought. Try to relive a very pleasant memory. You'll be surprised how well this works.

- A glass of milk just before bedtime can help you get to sleep. This is not just an old wives' tale. Milk contains the amino acid L-tryptophan, which has been known to induce sleep.

- Have a nice warm bath just before going to bed.

- Take a natural over-the-counter "sleep helper" vitamin supplement: copper, folic acid, vitamin B5, vitamin B12, vitamin B6, magnesium or calcium.

LACK OF EXERCISE

Physical exercise will improve general fitness as well as help you sleep. Even a short walk during the day can help. Regular exercise is even better. But don't do anything strenuous for the couple of hours prior to going to bed.

TOO MUCH WEIGHT

Obesity prevents people from being as active as they might want to be. Excess weight by itself can cause fatigue, and the physical stress that fat places on the body shortens life. If you have a lot of pounds to shed, don't be discouraged. Think in terms of a year and determine how much you need to lose each month to reach your goal. It's worth doing; and you'll sleep better, too.

NOT GETTING ENOUGH WATER

Adults lose about 3 quarts of water a day through evaporation, and more when they exercise. This liquid needs to be replaced, or they will become dehydrated. When that happens, they will feel sluggish and exhausted—and look it. In extreme cases, they might even pass out.

So on a normal day—you've heard this before—you must take in the equivalent of the water you've lost, which means drinking eight 8-ounce glasses of water or juice. That's

2 quarts. You will get the other quart from the food you eat. But, remember, if you're out in the heat or exercising, running or playing sports, you must drink more.

DEPRESSION

Sometimes a person can look or feel drained of energy because of depression. If you think you're depressed, or if the suggestions listed here don't work, see your doctor. He or she can prescribe medication and/or treatment that might change how you feel, improve your appearance and set you on a path toward a longer, healthier lifespan.

HORMONES

Hormonal imbalance can cause fatigue, especially in women in the early stages of menopause and beyond. Some women attribute being tired all the time to aging, but fatigue is not a function of age. Talk to your doctor.

NUTRITION FOR ENERGY

You cannot look and feel alive and energetic if you're not careful about your diet, making sure you're getting the vitamins and minerals you need. If you're not getting them from the food you eat, then add supplements, especially a good multivitamin.

You must have energy stored in your body in order to be able to use it, and that energy is glucose. The best source of glucose is carbohydrates. If you don't get enough carbohydrates, your body will use protein to get the glucose for energy, which will limit the building of muscle and the maintenance of bone, skin, hair and other tissue. Any glucose not needed right away gets stored as glycogen in the muscles and liver. Once the glycogen stores are filled up, any extra gets stored as fat.

FOR QUICK ENERGY, SIMPLE CARBOHYDRATES FROM FRUIT AND ENERGY DRINKS ARE GOOD SOURCES.

FOR MORE LASTING ENERGY, COMPLEX CARBOHYDRATES FROM WHOLE GRAIN BREADS, RICE, PASTA, CEREALS AND GRAINS WORK BEST.

ADDITIONAL TIPS

- Stick to a regular schedule of going to bed and getting up at the same time every day.

- Be consistent about taking naps. Take one every afternoon for no more than 20 minutes or none at all.

- Find the right room temperature for you and maintain it throughout the night.

- Do not eat heavily just before going to bed.

- When you cannot sleep at night, do your best to preserve your usual 24-hour cycle of activity, rest and exposure to light and dark. For example, do not get up, turn on bright lights and read or exercise. It is best to remain reclining in the dark and listen to music or an audio book.

HOME SPA FOR STRESS RELIEF

A medical doctor I know in New York City has a busy practice and typically stressful work days. When he comes home, he takes a bath without fail. He draws a tub of very warm water and soaks in it for about 20 minutes. I asked him why.

"When you get out of bed in the morning, your body's organs are more or less rested," he explained. "As the day goes on, those organs, as well as your mind and spirit, get put out of sorts due to the day's stressful wear and tear, as it were. Hydrotherapy, a 15- or 20-minute warm bath, relaxes me better than anything else I've tried. I can feel myself returning to a calm state, and I believe it is good for my long-term health and well-being, too."

Ever since he told me that, I have soaked in a relaxing tub of warm water every day I possibly can.

HYDROTHERAPY—AN ANCIENT HEALING PRACTICE

Hydrothermal therapy (hot water treatment) has been used as a traditional treatment for disease and injury by many cultures, including China and Japan. The ancient Greek healing god, Asklepios, advocated the use of water as medicine. Similarly, Roman physicians Galen and Celsus used therapeutic baths for many remedies. So, water therapy has been used for centuries to heal the sick.

A relaxing warm bath can help relieve congestion, aches and pains and will restore energy to your entire body, especially the neck and shoulders, which seem to suffer the most under stress.

By expanding your capillaries, the smallest blood vessels in the body, the warm water helps bring more blood to all your organs, providing them with more nourishment. Lying horizontally in a tub also relieves the heart from the burden of having to pump against gravity and increases blood flow.

One of the functions of your skin with its millions of pores is the elimination of toxins. Immersion in warm water for 15 or 20 minutes helps stimulate this process, causing perspiration, which in turn forces skin eruptions to emerge more quickly.

Scientific studies have proven that a warm tub bath has a positive effect on the nervous system. Warm water stimulates the nerve endings in your skin, which in turn deliver soothing messages to the organs, glands and muscles in your body.

Water therapy is also very effective as a non-toxic calming agent to soothe your body and help you get a better night's sleep. It acts as a mild tranquilizer if you do it just before going to bed. Taken in the morning, it provides energy for the day.

How to Set Up Your Home

Your peak of good health, ultimate beauty and youthful vitality can be attained only when your body, including your internal organs, mind and spirit are in harmony. But you don't have to go to a health spa, spend time in a whirlpool and indulge in a massage. An ordinary bathroom can be turned into a luxurious home treatment spa.

Here is a checklist of things you can do easily on your own to pamper yourself.

- Hang a "DO NOT DISTURB" sign on the bathroom door during every treatment—yes, I have one.

- Put your favorite plant or flower in the bathroom.

- Add a tranquil painting or 2.

- Soft towels—you deserve them.

- A soft bathroom mat.

- A tub tray, if you don't have enough shelf space close by.

- Soft, soothing music, if you wish—nothing loud, and no commercials.

- Something cool (not cold) to drink or sip with a straw. Cool juice is great.

- Have all your spa treatment products at arm's length:
  - Makeup cleanser/remover
  - Tissues
  - A rough or textured washcloth; a loofah or sponge is OK, too

ACHIEVE TOTAL RELAXATION

Most of us think we know when we are totally relaxed, but we usually aren't, not even when we're sleeping. Follow these 5 steps to make sure you are.

- Once your personal spa is ready, get into the bathtub and slowly sink into the water. Allow your shoulders to submerge up to your neck, even if you have to bend your legs and keep your knees out of the water. Make sure your feet are in the warm water, though. Now get comfortable. Get so comfortable that you do not have to hold up any part of your body. You must become "dead weight" to get totally relaxed.

- Focus your attention on one part of your body at a time and concentrate on relaxing it completely—you'll feel that part getting limp. Relaxing your back and neck muscles fully is most important. Rest your head on either a rolled-up towel, or better yet, a small waterproof head and neck cushion (you can buy one at most bath supply stores). It will greatly assist the relaxation process, and help keep your hair dry, as well.

- Once you are totally relaxed, take a half dozen or so deep breaths s-l-o-w-l-y, and then exhale completely.

- Think of one of the most pleasant things that ever happened to you. Focus on it.

- Now soak for 5 to 10 minutes, pretending you are asleep. Make sure your shoulders and the base of your neck remain immersed in the warm water. Your hydrotherapy treatment will do the rest.

To stay young you need to give yourself escape, time to be alone. A bath is a wonderful private place where you can relax and unwind your mind, body and soul, while revitalizing your spirit.

AFTERTHOUGHTS

Women are so busy today with plenty to be stressed out about. I can see it in their faces, so I know their bodies are paying a price, too. Occasionally, I try to talk one of my "stressed-out-take-a-quick-shower" friends into taking a breather and r-e-l-a-x-i-n-g while soaking in a warm tub of water, reminding her how great it would be for her body, as well as her mind. It's not easy to convey all the benefits, but once someone tries it, she usually finds a way to continue doing it.

I hope you will find a way to sit down, put your feet up and do nothing more often. Even a quiet 10 or 15 minutes of relaxation can heal your body for the moment. I often will sit in a comfortable chair for 10 minutes, my goal being to relax every muscle in my body. It's amazing how tense my muscles are when I first sit down, and how much looser after the 10 minutes.

CHAPTER 12

THE BEAUTY ORGASM

It's good for every cell in your body.

Sex is good for you in more ways than one. Yet in our society, there are many women conditioned to ignore this aspect of life. We must remember that not only is sex a God-given delight, but it is essential for the completion of a woman's personality and femininity. Sex is a necessary biological function, and orgasm is not only pleasurable, but a vital part of good health and beauty. I firmly believe that orgasms enhance a woman's beauty from the hair on her head to her toes.

Research has shown that in laboratory animals, regular mating leads to greater longevity and increases resistance to chemical and biological poisons, infections and strain. In some animals sexual intercourse is necessary for the optimal functioning of the endocrine system. In various parts of the body there are a number of important glands that form the endocrine system. They secrete hormones, which are chemical substances required for the chemical regulation of the body, some hormones actually being essential for life itself. There is considerable evidence that for animals, forced abstinence over long periods of time produces symptoms very much like human anxiety.

We know that tension and anxiety in human beings can lead to depression, lethargy and insomnia. But the physical results are even more insidious, because tension can lead to heart ailments, kidney dysfunction, high blood pressure, diabetes, arthritis, allergies and more.

If you're still not convinceed that orgasms can be helpful "preventive medicine," read on!

The Four Stages of Orgasm

Orgasm is a total physical response to the pleasure of lovemaking. In a very short span of time, a woman's body undergoes dramatic changes that are believed to make a contribution to overall physical health and beauty. Indeed, sexual hormones circulate to every part of her body from head to toe.

Orgasm can be obtained with a partner or be self-induced. Emotionally there is a difference, but for health and beauty purposes, it doesn't matter whether it occurs during intercourse or other forms of stimulation. Doctors have long used "therapeutic masturbation" to help a female overcome what is called "orgasm impairment." In all cases the physical climax is the same.

Dr. William Masters and Virginia Johnson, who did groundbreaking research on human sexuality, identified 4 stages of sexual fulfillment.

Excitement Phase

Before sexual excitement the sexual organs are in a resting state. As a woman becomes sexually aroused, the Excitement Phase begins. One of the first signs of sexual excitement in a woman is the presence of vaginal lubrication which comes from the walls of the vagina and is caused by a rise in the vaginal temperature.

As sexual excitement continues, blood accumulates in the pelvic area and sexual organs. The vagina expands and lengthens. The vaginal tissues begin to swell, along with the clitoris and breasts. At this point, the nipples sometimes begin to become erect. The muscles in the arms, legs, thighs and buttocks contract. Often a woman will also tense up the muscles in her abdomen as she tilts her pelvis up toward her mate (this is a learned response in some women, natural in others.) Probably her facial muscles are tensing up, too. All this is very much like a beautifully coordinated isometric exercise.

PLATEAU PHASE

As sexual excitement continues to build, the Plateau Phase is reached. The outer lips of the vagina become more swollen. The tissues of the walls of the outer third of the vagina, including the PC muscle (the pubococcygeal muscle, which controls the first third of the vagina), swell with blood and the vaginal opening becomes narrower.

The heart pumps blood faster, and breathing and pulse rate speed up. Many women also experience what doctors usually refer to as the sexual flush—a rosy, blush-like color over the skin of the face, neck and chest, as more blood and heat rise to the body's surface. At this point a film of perspiration can appear over some women's bodies.

ORGASMIC PHASE

As a woman moves into the Orgasmic Phase, breathing, pulse rate and blood pressure continue to rise. Increased muscle tension and blood supply to the sexual tissues reach a peak. Then, suddenly the PC muscle contracts rhythmically for a brief period. The muscles of the uterus and abdominal area contract, too, as does the hand and foot reflex, with a grasping muscular response. With the completion of the orgasm, everything—breathing, circulation and muscle tension, etc.—begins to return to normal.

RESOLUTION PHASE

Now the Resolution Phase begins. The sexual organs return to the resting position. The vagina shrinks back to its normal size. This may take only a few minutes or as long as half an hour. If orgasm has not occurred, the resolution phase can take 1 or 2 hours.

Altogether it's quite an extraordinary performance. This revving-up of circulation is much like the by-product of very effective physical exercise. But no other "exercise" is as natural as this or affects as many parts of the body at the same time; it also delivers the greatest number of beauty and health benefits. It's why so many women appear to glow when they're in love and enjoying a healthy sexual relationship. Orgasm helps you to achieve your highest level of individual beauty as it affects every part of your body, inside and out. Your complexion appears more youthfully radiant, your muscle tone improves, even your hair can look shinier.

Happily, this can happen at any age!

THE BENEFITS OF ORGASM

Sexual arousal involves the circulatory, respiratory, glandular and muscular systems throughout the entire body. It stimulates the endocrine system that regulates the body's chemistry through release of various hormones into the bloodstream.

These hormones are carried to virtually every part of the body, reaching the various organs, glands and tissues that will affect your health and beauty.

The endocrine glands play a very large part in your overall beauty. They affect the activity of every cell in the body, influence mental acuity, physical agility, build and stature, bodily hair growth, voice pitch, sexual urge and behavior. The endocrine system tempers every waking and sleeping moment of life and constantly modifies the way we feel, think, behave and react to all sorts of stimuli.

Orgasm stimulates the glands of the endocrine system, resulting in more hormones delivered to all parts of the body, nurturing its beauty and health.

BEAUTY AND HEALTH BENEFITS

THE SURFACE OF YOUR SKIN

Arteries and veins constricting in the pelvic area during orgasm affect the whole body. Many women experience a warm feeling over the enire surface of their skin as small blood vessels there relax and bring more blood and heat to the surface. This process is an excellent skin benefit because it promotes good circulation in the skin's outer layer and carries oil and moisture to the pores. This results in the skin acquiring a youthful, healthy glow. Moisture is also retained in the pores, preventing more rapid aging and leaving the surface of the skin soft and silky.

LUNGS

As the respiratory rate soars and excessive breathing becomes extremely deep and rapid—50 breaths per minute is a rate comparable to the most strenuous exercise. More oxygen is being brought into the body and the lungs are being used to their fullest capacity. Also, dangerous toxins are removed from the body with each deep exhalation.

Heart

Sexual activity speeds up the circulation, which affects the flow of blood, which in turn, affects the heartbeat. During orgasm the heart rate reaches 180 beats per minute, resulting in more of a workout than many other forms of exercise, such as jogging.

Hair

During the buildup of sexual excitement and orgasm, the accelerated heart rate pumping blood throughout the body at a much faster speed rushes the blood to the roots of the hair, feeding and nourishing them. If your head is lying flat on the bed, rather than propped up on a pillow or sitting up, your roots will benefit from an additional flow of blood.

Orgasm and Nutrition

The following vitamins and minerals are directly and indirectly involved in the production of hormones. In addition they contribute to the body's basic nutritional needs, which will help to create and maintain a healthy sexual appetite.

VITAMIN A IS REQUIRED FOR PRODUCTION OF THE SEX HORMONES.

B-COMPLEX VITAMINS AS A GROUP ARE MADE UP OF OVER 13 DIFFERENT VITAMINS, SEVERAL OF WHICH ARE NEEDED BEFORE SEX HORMONES CAN BE PRODUCED.

VITAMIN C PRODUCES MANY HORMONES THAT INFLUENCE YOUR SEX LIFE, INCLUDING A HORMONE THAT HELPS TO STIMULATE ORGASM.

VITAMIN E IS NEEDED FOR NORMAL SEX HORMONE PRODUCTION.

PHOSPHORUS HELPS NORMAL, HEALTHY FUNCTIONING OF THE SEXUAL NERVE CENTERS.

SODIUM AIDS MUSCLE CONTRACTION AND EXPANSION, AND NERVE STIMULATION.

POTASSIUM FACILITATES ENDOCRINE HORMONE PRODUCTION.

ZINC IS ESSENTIAL FOR THE GENERAL GROWTH AND PROPER DEVELOPMENT OF THE REPRODUCTIVE ORGANS.

ORGASMS AT ANY AGE

I first wrote about orgasm in 1977 in an article for Cosmopolitan magazine, and I've been asked questions about sex ever since. In the last 10 years, the most frequent question has been, "Can sex still be good when you get older?"

Most queries come from women younger than me who are worried that, at some point in their lives, they would have to "give it up!" I assured them that sex can be great at any age, provided you maintain your health. While it's true that intensity might change as we grow older, pleasurable sexual activity and orgasm and its benefits don't need to disappear.

One of the reasons women avoid sex is vaginal dryness, which can occur at any age for a variety of reasons, including stress, lack of foreplay, not allowing sufficient time for full arousal, hormonal changes and certain medications. Menopause and childbirth can interfere with normal vaginal lubrication, too.

Vaginal lubrication smoothes the way for sexual activity, helping to ensure that a woman's vaginal walls won't become irritated as the result of friction.

In older women, the Bartholin's glands, which generate lubricating fluid during sexual excitement, don't function as well or cease altogether.

There's a simple solution to vaginal dryness: Apply lubricant. There are many products available in drugstores and online without prescription.

- K-Y Jelly is the least expensive and most popular.

- Astroglide, a very good product, has a fun website, www.astroglide.com, where you can get a free sample.

- Replens, used with an applicator, lasts for three days, so you can be prepared and ready.

Each of these lubricants is water-based, water-soluble and pH-balanced to match normal body fluids. I do not recommend oil-based products, which can break down latex condoms; or petroleum-based lubricants that can provide a breeding ground for bacteria.

Another option is to consult your doctor to see if you're a candidate for an estrogen-based cream available by prescription.

Even if your Bartholin's glands are functioning well, there's nothing wrong with adding more lubrication for smoother action. Make it a fun part of foreplay and involve your partner.

FEMALE LIBIDO

There is no female Viagra—at least not yet, but there might be one day, since drug companies are trying hard to produce one. That's because 43% of women, compared to 31% of men, suffer some sort of sexual dysfunction.

Unfortunately, many women's natural embarrassment prevents them from speaking openly about the problem or seeking treatment. And some uninformed doctors dismiss it, sending their patients away with the suggestion that they simply have a glass of wine to relieve inhibitions.

If you think you might have a medical problem, I urge you to see a proper doctor. You not only deserve to enjoy that part of life, but also to become better-looking and healthier from it. If you wish to consult a specialist, these days all you need is a computer. Simply google "female pelvic medicine" and your city, and you will find a number of experts listed. Just make the call.

In the meantime, until the "pink" version of Viagra is developed, all claims of female herbal and hormone stimulants currently being marketed are scientifically unproven.

AFTERTHOUGHTS

Masters and Johnson were the first to study the anatomy and physiology of human sexuality. Their findings created much controversy at the time, but they helped correct the myths surrounding female sexuality and opened the door to the possibility that sex can be fun—and that it's not just an activity to be performed in the dark to make babies.

So today, unlike in generations past, words like women's libido, clitoris, labia, vulva, etc. can be spoken aloud and written about freely. And we now understand that anything consenting couples use in the bedroom—erotic film, vibrators, lubricants—is OK and desirable.

PART 3: LOOKING GOOD— FEELING GOOD

Never underestimate the power of looking and feeling good about yourself.

Have you ever noticed a stranger across a room, and for some reason you could not take your eyes off her? She might not have been a "raving beauty," as we say, or have had the best body in the world, but she was radiantly beautiful and commanded your admiration. You appreciate her pulled-together look and the confidence she exudes. You would like to know how she attained that aura. There are some people with innate instincts for looking great, but mostly it is a learned process.

It doesn't take a designer suit, diamonds on the fingers, the latest hairstyle or a fancy handbag to look fabulous. These things on their own do not always reflect good taste. A "perfect nose" and an "hourglass figure" aren't necessary either; nor do they guarantee attractiveness. What I'm talking about is looking good and feeling good with a confidence that "glows" and is admired by others.

I am talking about GLAMOUR!

So, what is glamour...what does it consist of? In a nutshell, it's looking and feeling your best with confidence. Can anybody be glamorous, no matter how old she is or what body type or skin color she has? Absolutely! These following chapters will tell you how.

CHAPTER 13

THE NO-MISTAKE MAKEUP SCHOOL FOR ALL AGES

Transform yourself into the beauty you really are.

In this chapter you will learn how to become skilled in the art of makeup for creating the most beautiful face you ever had...no matter your age. There are many things people do, or don't do, with makeup that prevents them from fully revealing their own special beauty. Many women confess that they don't know what to do—so they do nothing, or very little. Some even negate their natural beauty by applying makeup incorrectly, and are not even aware of it.

I will teach you how to accentuate your unique features, and de-emphasize what you may feel are your lesser attributes, and feel confident doing so...just as high fashion models do.

Many models are not beautiful in a classic sense, but they know how to make you think they are. They are skilled in the art of illusion, color and how to apply makeup to look their glamorous best. They have to be; their livelihood depends on it.

So, step into my world of ageless beauty and transform yourself with the look you always wanted—that of a beautiful, glamorous woman, and KNOW you look fantastic... you will!

PRODUCT CHOICES

Unflattering makeup is frequently a result of incorrect color choices, poor product consistency, inferior ingredients and/or the manner in which it is applied.

Simplicity in color will better serve your personal beauty. You do not need glitter, iridescence, "shiny stuff" or odd hues. The goal is to transform yourself, not become an advertisement for the latest makeup gimmick. Cosmetic companies are always developing the newest color, the latest lip gloss, or that must-have "something" to get your attention… and your money. Don't be impressed with fads and conjured-up trends—unless they make you look better. The only thing that should stand out on your face is your face.

In my heyday as a New York model, when I was being photographed for a well-known cosmetics company's ad, the makeup artist painted me with a bright blue eye shadow—one of that season's trendy colors. I was running late for my next job, a fashion shoot, and did not have time to wash it off. No sooner had I stepped through the door when the photographer, famous in that era, said, "Remove that awful blue eye shadow before getting on my set, please." It was not his idea of beauty, nor was it mine. I got rid of it immediately.

There are many colors and products that should not be used if you want to create an attractive, radiant look. One safeguard is to choose colors with a little earth tone in them. For example, a red lipstick could have a hint of brown or blue to keep it from looking like a bright orange red. Eye shadows should not be overly vivid or bright. Your eyes should steal the show, and with more natural colors, mascara and eyeliner, they will. Foundations and powders should more or less work with your own skin color—not too much red, yellow or orange, so that your lipstick, rouge and eye shadow won't clash. Powder can be a hint darker than your skin color, if you like, but the same color is good, too.

ACCENTUATE YOUR HIGHLIGHTS, STRENGTHS AND UNIQUE FEATURES

PREPARATION

How your makeup looks toward the end of the day depends partly on how you clean and prepare your skin at the beginning No matter what you use to cleanse your face and neck, always use a toner/astringent afterward. It's best to apply it with a thin washcloth; its texture will help get into your pores, remove residual oils and bacteria, and prepare your skin to absorb all the nutrients from the day cream you need to apply next. (Remember, inexpensive, thin, white washcloths are available at most discount department stores.)

The day cream you apply under any makeup base should not be oily. Use one that absorbs into the skin to nourish and protect it all day. After you're finished, wait a second or 2, and then lightly wipe your face and neck to remove any excess. Only then will you be ready for your makeup base.

FOUNDATION

The purpose of a foundation is not only to make your skin look beautiful and its color even, but also to prevent drying out from the sun, wind, and indoor heat or air conditioning, which ages the skin faster. The protective layer of foundation helps block this damage. But don't confuse foundation with sunblock, needed for full protection when exposing the skin directly to the sun for sports or on the beach.

The only makeup base that is light in texture, easy to apply, blends evenly on the skin, has a wonderful consistency, yet covers well is a liquid "oil/water" blend. Such a formula is good for all types of skin—dry, normal or oily—because it prevents the foundation product from settling into lines and wrinkles, making them appear deeper than they really are.

Your foundation color should be about the same color as your skin. A darker base will settle into the pores making them and any facial lines or wrinkles look more prominent as the day goes by. The color tone should be neutral in order to make your skin appear natural and not compete with other makeup colors. It's the beginning—the base—for the total look of delicate beauty.

HOW TO APPLY FOUNDATION

It is best not to use fingers, which are warm, because they tend to open up the pores more, causing the foundation to sink deeper. Also, it is much more difficult to achieve an even finish on your face using fingers. Use a sponge. Be sure to cover the skin right up to and under the eyes, as well as the inside corners of the eyes by the nose. Many women miss these corners where the skin is often darker and needs covering to even it out for a more youthful appearance.

Do not apply foundation on eyelids, however. It will cause your eye shadow to smudge, may very well change the eye shadow's color, and will prevent it from going on evenly.

Don't forget the front of the neck. This accomplishes 2 things: It evens out the skin color to match your face, and it protects the skin of the neck from the elements.

After a second or two, remove any excess base on your skin, using a tissue and brushing it ever-so-lightly over the entire face and neck. Later, you will powder over the foundation to give it a "matte" finish and create a soft, angelic look. Any shine left on the face makes lines and wrinkles look more obvious. To test this, take a mirror and stand at a window sideways before you powder. See how the shine plays up any lines and wrinkles. Then apply powder and see how they soften and almost disappear.

Eye Makeup

Everyone needs eye makeup—I have never known a model who was not asked to wear eye makeup for a shoot, even if you could not tell by looking through the lens. All types of eyes can be made to look fascinating and beautiful—small, large and deep-set eyes, even eyes that seem too close together—so long as you master the artistry involved.

If you are not accustomed to eye makeup, be sure you experiment with it before a big event: You don't want to rush it while you are learning. Once learned, a routine for your particular type should be simple and quick for you.

How to Apply Mascara

Water and smudge-proof mascara is the best for obvious reasons. Either black or brown will give anyone a soft, glamorous look.

Before applying, make sure you remove any trace of oil or cleanser from your eyelashes, eyelids and under your eyes, using a tissue or thin washcloth and a toner/astringent; otherwise, even the best mascara might smudge during the day. Use an eyelash curler to create a more open and dramatic look Apply one coat of mascara, then go back and apply a second coat. Don't forget the bottom lashes too—that's a must! Make sure your lashes do not stick together in clumps. They must be separated. A good mascara brush should automatically do this…if some lashes stick together, separate them carefully with a toothpick.

FALSE EYELASHES? YOU BET! TRY THEM!

I know, you don't wear them because you don't know how, or which type or color to use, or you have seen some that look ridiculous and you don't want to look like "that." Or you are one of the lucky few that don't need them. I am the mistress of false eyelashes. I have been known to say, "I'd rather be seen without my lipstick than without my false eyelashes." It's true! I have them on in all of my pictures over the past 50 years. Can you tell? Be honest.

The hardest part is to find the false lashes that look natural, not too thick and not too thin, but just right. False lashes look real if they have soft hair, are flexible and have a clear base strip that makes them unnoticeable when worn. My manicurist of 10 years never knew I had them on until I called attention to them. They are fun, alluring and they do make you look younger.

How to Apply False Eyelashes

First you must prepare your false lashes.

If your lashes are too wide: Lift one eyelash out of the box. Holding it with both hands at the ends, place it up to your eyelid next to your own lashes. In most cases, it will be too wide for your eyes. (I always have to trim the width.) Snip off a few hairs at one end and test it again. Now trim the other eyelash to match. When cut and applied correctly, no one will even know you have them on.

If your lashes are too long: Trim the length—but not too much. You can always go back and do more. Point the end of the scissors into the tips of the eyelashes and snip. Do not cut straight across in one swoop; they look more natural when uneven.

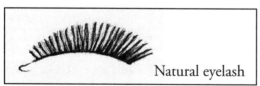 Natural eyelash
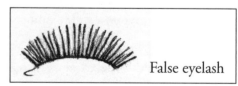 False eyelash

Notice how your natural eyelashes look in relation to your nose. So trim the false eyelash the same way—shorter toward the nose and a little shorter in general if you like. Also make a little snip on the outside end to round it off a little.

Make sure all oil is off your eyelids. Use a toner/astringent with a tissue or a thin washcloth, as I mentioned before. Mascara your natural eyelashes (top and bottom) before applying the false ones…they will blend in better.

Now apply eyelash glue on the clear strip—you don't need much. Some people squeeze the tube directly on the strip part. I put a little glue on my vanity table or on the top of a jar of cream, then pick some up with a toothpick and place it on the strip. (Whichever method is most comfortable for you is fine.) Now, with both hands holding the lash, place it next to your own lashes. Use tweezers to pull it to one side or the other, as needed. If you do this immediately, before the glue dries, it will be very easy to adjust. (You will have about a minute.) Don't worry about getting the eyelashes off. When ready, and if necessary, just put a drop or 2 of water on the base strip, and they can be removed easily.

After applying both false lashes, blend your natural lashes into them. Do this with your fingers or a small eyelash or eyebrow brush. You want them to look as one.

How to Clean False Eyelashes

Place them on a counter and put a few drops of water over them. After a minute or so the glue will be easy to pull off the clear strip with your fingers. Let dry and they will be ready to wear again. You can also place the lashes between tissues; wrap the tissue around a pencil to let dry or store them.

I often sleep with mine on. Since I take tub baths (rather than showers), they stay dry, so I leave them on when I cleanse my face at night and climb into bed. Occasionally I find one on the pillow in the morning or in my hair. When that happens, I simply clean it and put it back on (or get a fresh pair)!

How to Apply Eyeliner

I don't believe in black eyeliner except for African Americans with a dark shade of skin color, and maybe for a few who use it v-e-r-y lightly; otherwise the look is too heavy and harsh. You will find dark brown and charcoal work much better for most.

The "lead" of an eyeliner pencil should glide over the skin without pulling it and go on easily. It should be just soft enough so that, instead of having to use a pencil sharpener to keep it pointed, you can firmly pinch the tip and hold it a few seconds to elongate it between your fingers. Save the sharpener only for when absolutely necessary.

When using an eyeliner pencil, if you have to pull your eyelid taut in order to apply an eyeliner pencil, it usually means the pencil's "lead" is too hard. It is normal, however, to hold the eyelid on one side so that it stays in place while applying eyeliner.

You can start at either corner of the eyelid, but make sure you color the entire width of the lid. Applying eyeliner all the way toward the nose gives the eyes a softer, more open look, but make it light and thin. You can smudge the eyeliner ever so slightly, if you like. This gives the eyes a softer look rather than a heavy dark line.

If you are wearing false lashes, follow the same instructions as above. Just continue the eyeliner a little past the false lashes toward the nose.

For the lower lid, be sure to apply the eyeliner lightly. Do NOT go too close to the nose—stop about 1/3 of the way in from the nose. Apply it wider and a little darker as you get to the outside corner.

Eyebrow Pencil

Have you ever glanced at someone from across the room and, before you noticed anything else about them, you saw 2 black "lines" above their eyes? Well I have, and I've seen even worse! I don't know why, but for some reason, American women seem to mess up their eyebrows more than women in other countries.

Eyebrows are modifiers, eye beautifiers. They exist to complement and enhance the look of the eyes. They should act as a frame for the specific shape and type of your eyes, not overpower the face or draw attention to themselves.

Look at classic paintings by masters like Rembrandt, Renoir, Rubens and da Vinci (forget about the Mona Lisa, though!). Note that these great painters treated the eyebrows of their women with understatement and as an accompaniment

Difficulty with proper eyebrow shape and color is often the result of focusing on the eyebrows per se, rather than on how they can be most flattering to the shape of a person's eyes and face. When you finish defining your eyebrows, step back from the mirror and look at your face from a distance. Do your eyebrows look overpowering or too dark for your face? Or are they too pale? Are they symmetrical?

How to Apply Eyebrow Pencil

The consistency of the "lead" is most important for a great-looking eyebrow. If it's too hard, the pencil does not adhere to the skin well; if it's too soft, it's all but impossible to get a delicate-looking eyebrow. Use short, light strokes for each "hair," allowing them to blend together. Feathering your pencil strokes with an upward and outward motion will make them look like your own hair (provided you powder lightly over them as explained below). Never draw the pencil through the whole eyebrow in one stroke. To make my eyebrows even more natural-looking, I add a few strokes with a darker colored pencil for contrast.

As for color, choose an eyebrow pencil that matches or takes on the color of your hair. Never use black, even if your hair is black, unless you are African-American and have very dark skin.

EYEBROW TIPS

To make your eyes appear larger and more open, make sure your eyebrows don't "sit" low over your eyes. Instead, keep sufficient space between them by plucking clean from underneath the brows. But not too much, or it will make them too thin. If you have bushy eyebrows, you might need to trim the tops to keep the length short and to make them look thinner.

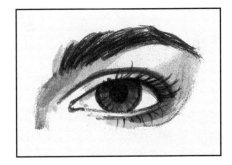

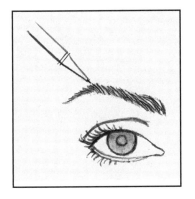

The shape of your eyebrows should be in a slight arch, wider toward your nose and thinning toward the temples. The peak of the arch should generally be about 3/4 of the distance of the width of your eye toward the temple.

Begin your eyebrows about where your eyes begin inside your nose, and end them just beyond where your eyes end toward your temples.

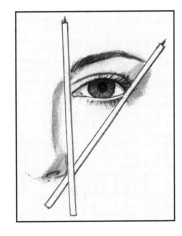

If your eyes are too close together, start the eyebrow a little further from your nose, creating a slightly larger space between your eyebrows than normal. Not too great a space, though, just enough to give a more open look, maybe 1/16 to 1/8 of an inch across. Step back and see if it's too much.

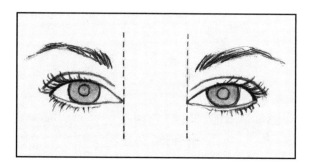

USING POWDER

Once the eyebrows are completed, powder over them lightly against the direction of the eyebrow hair. This will them give a softer, natural look. Then, with 2 fingers, brush upward toward the forehead and nose to remove excess powder and restore the hair to its natural position. You could buy an eyebrow brush for this purpose, but your fingers are just as effective—and faster.

EYE SHADOW

Eye shadow should be worn to enhance the type and shape of your eyes. You should never wear a bright or iridescent color that stands out like a Christmas bulb! It's the beauty of the entire face that is important. Choose colors that enhance the face, or seem to change the shape of the eye, if desired. A blue, iridescent eyelid will not get the job done! My recommendation is a matte eye shadow with high pigment for longer lasting color throughout the day.

HOW TO APPLY EYE SHADOW

I apply eye shadow before applying foundation. Often powdered eye shadow falls onto the foundation, and then needs to be removed. I have found it's easier to simply apply the eye shadow first and then put on the foundation, thus eliminating the problem.

When you're ready, remove all oil from the upper eyelids as well as the eyelashes. Doing so helps the eye shadow stay in place, and it will be less likely to crease or smudge. Powdered eye shadow should be applied with a tiny sponge or a small, narrow, blunt eyeliner brush.

First, apply an off-white or light beige eye shadow on the eyelid itself. Do not go above the eyelid crease with the light color. Next, put on a darker eye shadow above the crease.

MAKING EYES LOOK LARGER

Apply an off-white eye shadow on the upper eyelid, bringing it all the way to the inside corner next to the nose. For dark skin colors, use a color several shades lighter than your natural skin tone. Apply a darker eye shadow in and above the eye socket. Bring it down and around to the outside corner and into the bottom of the eye about 1/3 of the way, tapering off in the bottom lashes. Now bring the dark shadow in toward the nose on the upper lid, but not as wide. Make sure you smudge the edges using a tissue or your finger so there are no hard lines of demarcation.

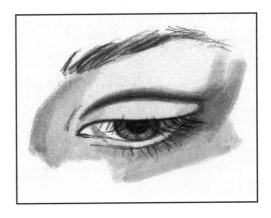

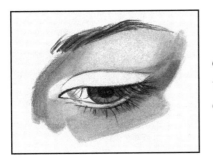

For dark eyelids or deep-set eyes, apply off-white eye shadow from the inner corners of the upper lids to the outside corners. For dark skin colors use a color several shades lighter than your natural skin tone.

For heavy or prominent eyelids, apply a dark eye shadow on the upper eyelids. You also might try a lighter shade on top of that above the eyelid.

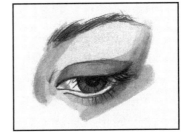

For eyes that are too close together, apply off-white eye shadow on the inner 1/3 corners of the eyelids up to the nose to give the illusion of a wider pair of eyes. Again, for darker skin colors use a color several shades lighter than your natural skin tone.

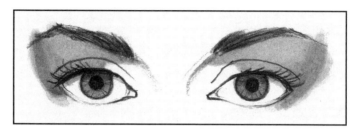

HIGHLIGHT

Using highlight under the eyes to hide dark circles or discoloration will make your face appear more youthful and softer-looking. This takes very little time once you have done it a couple of times. You can get highlight that is lightweight yet hides dark circles and discoloration well. Purchase one that is several shades lighter than your natural skin or foundation color to offset the discoloration under your eyes. The one many models use is made with mica and bismuth oxychloride, ingredients that "reflect" light from dark areas, providing lightweight camouflage that is not noticeable, yet does the job.

HOW TO USE HIGHLIGHT

Apply very small amounts of highlight to any dark area of the face. Carefully blend into the skin or foundation. (The best effect is achieved by applying highlight over foundation.) Use a makeup brush or small makeup sponge to thin out and blend the edges to remove any lines of demarcation. Now powder over. The powder will camouflage and blend the highlight for a very natural look.

HIGHLIGHT TIPS

Camouflage a more prominent chin
Apply highlight along the jawbone from ear to ear. Blend into foundation so there is no demarcation line. The famous model, Wilhelmina, did this and she had 27 Vogue magazine covers to her name!

Soften smile lines

With the tip of a small makeup sponge, place a small amount of highlight in the creases of your smile lines. Use a finger or sponge to gently smudge. Powder over and it will blend in. If it doesn't, you used too much.

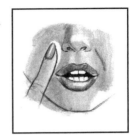

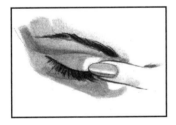

Hide dark circles under the eyes

Apply highlight evenly and sparingly in the dark areas under the eyes. It's best to use a small makeup brush or small sponge with a "corner." You can put it directly on the skin itself after moisturizer, or over your foundation. Whichever you do, make sure you powder over lightly. This "sets" the highlight, keeps it from settling into fine lines and gives it a more natural, finished appearance.

De-emphasize frown lines

Place highlight in frown lines as above and follow the same instructions as above for softening smile lines.

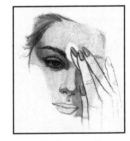

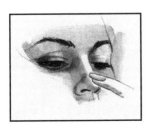

Widen eyes

As with eye shadow, applying highlight to the inner 1/3 corners of the eyelids up to the nose gives the illusion of a wider pair of eyes.

Lengthen low forehead or make face longer

Apply highlight along the hairline and blend downward about an inch or so.

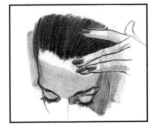

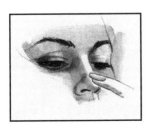

Correct a flat nose

Apply highlight down the center of the nose. Use very little, keeping if off the sides of the nose. Smooth and blend down center. Powder over. Do not leave a harsh line of white—it should not be obvious.

ROUGES

Applying rouge is often misunderstood. I'm setting the record straight for you! Whether you use cream or powder rouge, the rules for putting them on are the same.

CREAM ROUGE

Cream rouge, usually applied with a fingertip or 2, glides over the skin smoothly and goes exactly where you want it to. It can be used over foundation or directly on the skin. It gives a soft, even glow, and its edges are easy to taper or blend to make it appear natural. Never use rouge with glitter or sparkles. If you are over 20, it will make your skin appear older and, if I may say so, a bit tacky. Only natural-looking colors should be worn—no odd colors. Remember, you are the star.

Never use rouge to change the shape or contour of your face. Rather, let it create a natural, beautiful glow on your cheeks. Then add just a touch on your forehead hairline, and a bit on your neck—to blend face and neck. If you have never tried this, you will be amazed at the look. You also must blend edges, so you cannot see where the rouge ends.

Pat one finger in rouge pan, then smudge it around slightly on the palm of your other hand so that the rouge is thinned out on your finger. You need very little, and this helps keep you from putting on too much.

Lightly tap cream rouge on cheeks, putting less rouge toward the temples and nose and more toward the center of the cheeks. Lightly blend the rouge up and over as well as down and under the cheekbones. Now smooth it out toward the temples and nose, leaving a little more color toward the center of the cheek. Blend carefully so you cannot see where the rouge stops.

A model's trick for a softer, more natural appearance is to dab some rouge on the tip of your chin, the center of your neck, and a few spots on your forehead along the hairline. Blend these areas so you see only a hint of color, smoothing the forehead rouge into the hairline, and spreading it around on the neck and bottom edge of the chin.

POWDER ROUGE (POWDER BLUSHER)

Why is powder rouge necessary when you have already used a cream rouge? Well, cream rouge is applied under powder. It blends smoothly onto the skin or into the skin foundation and stays on all day. You cannot adjust or add cream rouge once you've powdered your face. Sometimes, during the day, I take a quick look in the mirror and feel I need a touch more color. So I get out my trusty powder rouge and give it a quick brush up. Powder rouge is also great to add more color for evening wear, when you might need a little extra. Do not use powder rouge with iridescence in it, as the shine actually will heighten wrinkles and skin imperfections. Soft, muted colors will be more flattering.

Use a soft, clean makeup brush anywhere you have applied the cream rouge. Anytime you feel you need a little more color, just brush a little on.

Don't forget to wash your brush. It really helps the blusher go on evenly.

Powder

Powder should be light in weight and fine so that you can blend the foundation, cream rouge and highlight together. There should be no "shine" or glitter in the formula, as it will emphasize skin imperfections and make even small lines and wrinkles more obvious.

I have always worn powder. It sets my foundation and cream rouge to stay on for the day and evening. It helps keep my own natural moisture in and helps protect my skin against sun damage.

How to camouflage large pores

Apply foundation using a color no darker than the shade of your skin, then tissue off excess. With plenty of powder on the puff, gently press it into the skin. Do not rub the puff across the skin. When you have powdered your entire face, brush the puff very lightly over the top of the skin to remove the excess. What remains will cover the skin while leaving enough in the pores to camouflage them. (A powder with a shine would cause the pores to show more prominently.) Keep extra powder puffs around for when the one you're using starts to look matted down.

Lip Makeup

It's okay to simply slap a little lipstick on if you are not going anyplace special, but for important occasions you'll want your most glamorous "movie star" lips—no matter the size or type of lips you have.

LIPSTICK

Choose a non-greasy lipstick for longer wear. I recommend colors with earth tones in them—they are more flattering. For example, an orange that has a little blue or brown mixed in will still be orange, but is a softer color for your face. And please, no tacky iridescence or glitter in it!

LIP LINER PENCIL

The consistency of the "lead" in a lip liner pencil makes or breaks the look of the lips. If it's too hard, it pulls the lips, making it difficult to outline them and have the color blend in with your choice of lipstick color. If it's too soft, you cannot control where the color goes. Your lip line will look "feathered"—exactly what you want to avoid.

LIP GLOSS

A subtle lip gloss can add beauty to your lips. A greasy-looking mouth, however, is not glamorous. Apply the gloss only on the lower lip but not on the lip line itself. Lip gloss can also be worn alone to keep your lips moist and soft throughout the day.

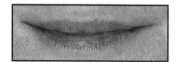
Pre-makeup lips

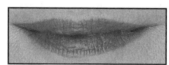
After using lipstick

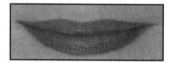
After using
"fuller lips" technique

LIPSTICK, LINER AND GLOSS FOR FULLER LIPS

Follow these step-by-step instructions using model makeup tricks. They are not difficult to master and can result in a very glamorous and alluring look.

- Apply lipstick using your full lip line. Blot lightly.

- Again, the consistency of the lip liner pencil is very important—not too hard or too soft. Make sure the pencil has a sharp enough point. Then lightly blend the liner around the edges of your lips and into the lipstick, making sure to cover the full edge of your lip line. Even go slightly over your lip line. Do not just draw a dark line around the lips. With your pencil, smudge or blend the 2 colors together so there is no distinct line of demarcation between the lipstick and lip pencil.

- If you want or need to add more lipstick, now is the time to do it. For fuller looking lips you can apply a lighter shade of lipstick on the inside of your lower lip. If you do, take care not to go onto or over the lip line with this second color. It would spoil the fuller lips effect you have just created.

- Blot your lips and powder lightly over the edges of your lip line. The powder covers up your secret method of achieving fuller lips; leaving a shine on the outside edges of your lipstick only makes your secret obvious, so, again—no shine on the lip line itself.

- If you are going to wear lip gloss, now is the time to put it on; but only on the inside lower lip. Do not apply it on the lip line itself; you will expose your fuller lip secret!

Note: *If your lips are full or wide, you can use the same 5 steps, but bring the lipstick and lip pencil just inside the lip line.*

Special Tips

Quick Overall Makeup Check—A Must

So you finish your makeup, and take one last check in the mirror—the same mirror you just used to apply your makeup…right? Wrong! Since lighting varies in different places, it's best to take a quick check in a different mirror, preferably with different lighting, especially for when you want to make sure everything is perfect. There have been times that I looked in a different mirror and found that I had on too much rouge, or my lipstick seemed too dark for the dress. But that is what quick checks are for.

Achieving a High Cheekbones Look

Prominent cheekbones are important in the high fashion modeling world. I was born with very high cheekbones and hated them in my younger years. It wasn't until I went to New York to model that I began to like them. All high fashion models learn how to create the illusion of high cheekbones if they don't have them naturally. And if they already have them, they make them even more pronounced for certain ads.

They use shading cream, which comes in a thick cream or powder blusher form. To achieve the look of high cheekbones, the color must be several shades darker than your skin or foundation color.

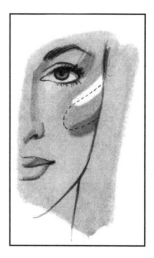

- Apply cream shading with your fingers or small sponge below the cheekbone and apply rouge in the middle of it. For an even more pronounced look, add highlight above the cheekbone. If you use a powder blusher shading, follow the same rules using a soft blusher brush.

- Make sure to blend edges—you do not want to see where shading begins or ends. If you have added too much shading, powdering over will help soften the look.

- Step back from the mirror and take a look from a few feet away to see if you have overdone it. If not, then powder down over it all and watch it blend in to become your "very real" high cheekbones.

How Safe Is Permanent Makeup?

I have seen successful permanent makeup that looks good. When this is the case, and there are no problematic side effects, people are very happy with it.

Start with understanding the risks of the procedure, researching the process and finding the most capable person to do the artwork. It is very important to make sure you understand and use proper care to reduce the risks after the procedure, too. However, sometimes even this is not always enough to prevent problems.

Many permanent makeup "artists," although they might be technically proficient, are not really artists. I have seen harsh dark "lines" for eyebrows—not feathered at all—and some that did not match the shape of the eyes or face. Another example could be lips done in an unbecoming color. These are some of the things that have to be considered as potential dangers.

If you decide you want permanent makeup, look for a practitioner (in a cosmetic surgeon's office) who has done the procedure for several years. These people, who are often registered nurses (this should be verified by you), must work under the direction of the doctor for safety. Talk with them or, better yet, meet one or 2 of their patients, and study the personal portfolio of their work. If there is no personal portfolio, look elsewhere.

Here are just some issues to consider in regard to permanent makeup before planning a procedure.

- **Blood-born diseases.** If the equipment used is contaminated, it is possible to contract diseases like hepatitis B and C, tetanus and tuberculosis. The fact that blood banks require a 12-month waiting period after the procedure before allowing a person to donate blood says a lot!

- **Allergic reactions.** Injected dyes can cause allergic skin reactions, resulting in an itchy rash, which may keep recurring for years after the procedure.

- **Scarring.** If you are prone to developing keloids (scars that grow beyond normal boundaries), the last place you want to see one is on your face!

- **Redness and swelling.** Permanent makeup procedures can lead to local bacterial infections, producing redness and swelling.

- **Removal of permanent makeup.** Removing permanent makeup is a painstaking process. It usually takes several treatments and is expensive. Complete removal without scarring may be impossible.

If permanent makeup is done under the proper circumstances and by a qualified practitioner, preferably a registered nurse in a doctor's office, there is an excellent chance you will be fine. I considered having my eyebrows done at one time, but discarded the idea in favor of performing the artwork myself every day.

Whatever decision you make, I urge you to take the steps necessary to ensure your safety before going forward.

AFTERTHOUGHTS

At the beginning of this chapter I suggested that if you followed my suggestions, you will look in the mirror and "know" you're glamorous, having enhanced your natural beauty by creating your very own secret illusions. I bet you will also spot a head or two turning when you're out and about. This proves you did a great job! You may even carry yourself with a new "glow" you've never had before. I have been around beautiful women since my earliest modeling days. I have seen them before and after makeup; and I know myself before and after. You bet you can do it, too!

CHAPTER 14

A MORE PERFECT FIGURE

Learn to fool the eye,
no matter what your body type.

Nobody's perfect! Not even the most glamorous, beautiful women, including models and actresses. Everyone has some kind of figure flaw or 2—shoulders too narrow, hips too wide, neck too short or too long, bust too small or too large, short legs—the list goes on and on. This chapter will tell you how to conceal your weak points, make the most of your strong points, and "improve" your figure, creating a picture of total attractiveness with grace and style.

You will learn the art of figure illusion—yes, it can be learned. We've all done a little of it by trial and error. The "beautiful, glamorous people" have done it for years. Remember Jamie Lee Curtis in More magazine having the courage to show herself in bra and panties with all of her physical flaws prominently on display, but a page later looking fantastic in a dress?

Remember that your appearance talks before you open your mouth. The success of your appearance depends first on knowing your figure flaws, then camouflaging them and balancing them with your strong traits. Money is not the most important factor here. It can buy expensive clothes, but not figure know-how or good taste.

The undeniable fact is that clothes—one of a woman's greatest allies in presenting herself—are often responsible for creating precisely the opposite effect. Many women admit they are not sure of the best way to dress for their body type, what hairstyle looks best or how much jewelry to wear with an outfit.

Well, look around and you will see what NOT to wear: Oversized clogs or platforms in which someone stumbles along, shoes with open heels that noisily clonk with every footstep, outlandish hairstyles, clashing colors and designs poorly suited for a particular figure type, etc. The well-to-do depend on designer creations to give them "style"—and even then it's not always the right style for them. After all, the designer just wants to show off the dress. So you need to see the total complete picture of your body and learn to judge for yourself.

You can balance your figure even if you're terribly overweight by choosing the best styles, fabrics, colors and accessories for you.

I wear shoes with at least a one-inch heel in order to give the illusion of balance between my legs and torso; otherwise my torso would look slightly elongated. I also avoid hip huggers, since they make my legs look just a bit short. Slacks at my natural waistline with shoes with at least a one-inch heel give me a well-proportioned look.

Your Proportions

Before you can present your figure at its best you must take an honest look at the problems and the potential of your own image or silhouette. Only when you know them, can you do something about them.

A simple way to tell if you are overweight, if scales scare you, is to subtract your waist measurement from your height in inches, without shoes, and if the result is 36 or greater, you are not too heavy. For example, 5' 7" converted to inches is 67. Subtract a 24-inch waist. Since the result, 43, is higher than 36, the woman in question is not overweight. This formula won't apply to professional athletes, who carry a lot of extra muscle.

Don't forget that the length of the various parts of your body also plays an important role in the picture you present. For perfect proportions, the distance from the pelvic bone to the bottom of the feet, standing, should be equal to the distance from the top of the head to the pelvic bone. If the measurement from the pelvic bone down to the feet is more than 1 and 1/2 inches shorter than the top measurement, you are probably short-legged.

A simple test for short-waistedness is to look at the length of the arms. Let your arms hang down at your side by your thighs. If your wrist bone is lower than your coccyx bone (your tailbone, the last vertebra on your spine) by more than 1 and 1/2 inches, you are probably short-waisted and must compensate.

CORRECT WAY TO MEASURE YOUR BODY

It's a good idea to measure parts of your body from time to time—perhaps every 6 months or once a year—and keep a record for comparison. You'll find it interesting to refer to over the years. It also will enable you to monitor any changes and, if necessary, take corrective action by spotting problems early. The measurements should be done the same way each time.

Measure each part of your body listed below and fill in the blanks. Take them with your usual underwear on, since you are preparing to balance your figure when dressed. Use a flexible measuring tape, holding it snugly, but not tightly, around these 9 key areas.

Neck _____

Upper arm _____

Bust _____

Waist _____

Hips _____

Upper thigh _____

Mid-thigh _____

Calf _____

Ankle _____

HOW TO MEASURE EACH PART

Neck: Place the tape around the middle of the neck.

Upper arm: Place the tape 4 inches down from the armpit.

Bust: Place the tape over the fullest part of the bust and straight across the back.

Waist: Measure your natural waistline, the smallest part. Don't hold your breath.

Hips: Measure about 7 inches below the natural waistline on short figures, 9 inches below on tall ones.

Upper thigh: Place the tape as high as possible and pull it around your leg.

Mid-thigh: Measure halfway between the upper thigh and the knee.

Calf: Measure around the largest part of the calf.

Ankle: Place tape around the part just above the anklebone.

GET THE FACTS RIGHT

It's a good idea to be aware of all your measurements, but another big help is to see the image of your body in outline.

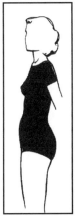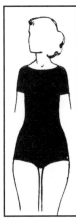

The easiest way is to have a friend take a black and white picture of you wearing a swimsuit and your usual hairdo, from the front, back and side. Be sure to show your full body from head to toe.

With a piece of tracing paper, draw the silhouette, and you will see the outline of your overall image.

Having the side as well as front and back views will graphically point out that measurements alone do not tell the story. Each figure has individual differences of width versus depth of various parts of the body, which may add or detract from our appearance.

For example, if your silhouette looks like the one shown here, it's obvious that your hips are larger than your shoulders and you may want to balance the hips with the shoulders for a "more perfect figure."

LEARN TO SEE YOURSELF AS OTHERS SEE YOU

You have all heard the timeless expression, "First impressions are the most important." Studies have shown that people make snap judgments within a few seconds after meeting someone. Your appearance gives others clues to your personality, social status, and occupation, and even what you might expect out of life. As unfair as this may seem to people who emphasize the importance of inner beauty, we happen to live in a world that dwells on initial, superficial outside impressions.

There's a word for it, derived from the German: gestalt. It means a "unified whole, a configuration, pattern, or organized field having properties that are greater than the sum of its component parts." The image of a person is created by how her individual traits all fit or work together, and by how she shows her awareness of her appearance in the form of poise, carriage and posture. A woman can have expensive jewelry, an exquisite hairstyle and the most up-to-date, chic lothing; each element in itself could be striking, but together they could look incongruous and unflattering.

So how do we go about making sure everything about the whole works? There is one simple rule: first the outfit, then the detail.

CHECK YOURSELF OUT

Begin by consulting your best friend. No, not your girlfriend, but a full-length mirror. Used properly, it will be your truest confidante. Be sure it is a full-length mirror that shows everything at once. When you are dressed, stand at least 5 feet away and take a critical look at yourself. What total image do you present to the world? Should you make your hair a little fuller to balance your fuller figure? Would it be better if your clothing hugged your hips more to balance with your shoulders? Are your clothes the right length? Do all the colors go well to-

> NO MATTER HOW BEAUTIFUL A PART OF THE WHOLE IS, IT IS THE WHOLE THAT MUST LOOK BEAUTIFUL.

gether? Are you wearing too many accessories? If you are not sure, remove some of them and take another look. You shouldn't add so much as a necklace without checking it out in a mirror as a part of the whole, if you really want to look your best.

Learning to criticize yourself at home is no different than criticizing another woman's appearance, which we do all the time without even thinking.

One way to take an honest look at your silhouette is to face the mirror with light coming only from behind you. You will see what others see. It's an excellent test—try it! Also, use a hand mirror to examine your back and side "profiles." If you are accustomed to checking only your front view, you may be surprised. Food for thought!

BALANCING YOUR TOP WITH YOUR BOTTOM—IF YOU NEED IT

Models, whose careers depend on their "perfect" figures, have legs that are too long or too short for their bodies, heads too small for their bodies, shoulders too narrow, and bosoms too large or too small. But they all look beautiful and most "appear" perfect because they have learned from studies in the mirror and their own photos what their shortcomings are and how to disguise them.

Let's look at 6 common problems of proportion balancing.

1. LONG-WAISTED (Shorter legs with longer body)

CAN WEAR

- waistbands slightly higher than your waist. Half an inch or an inch can make a big difference. You can do this by moving your belt up a little or simply pulling the garment up slightly to just above the waistline. No one but you can tell exactly where your real waist is located unless you have on a bikini. When you buy pants, skirts and dresses, pick out garments that have just the right height waistband for you; for example a waistband that sits lower on your hips will make your legs seem shorter and your torso longer. You'll soon get used to the feeling of the waistband being a little higher than normal.

- soft tops with an undefined waistline.

- wide belts, sashes, and wide, horizontally designed fabric belts (if you are slim).

- long dresses and skirts (with the higher-than-normal waistband mentioned above). This gives the illusion of longer legs and a more flowing line between waistband and feet.

- skirts and dresses near the knee. This helps make the space between waist and knee longer than it is.

SHOULD AVOID

- clinging tops.

- small, narrow belts at regular waistline, loose low waistlines of any kind.

- hip huggers (pants made with the waistband at least 2 inches below your waistline). They make your legs look shorter, which in turn makes your torso look even longer.

- above-the-knee skirts or shorts.

2. SHORT-WAISTED (Long legs with short midriff)

CAN WEAR

- hats with height or an upward sweep.
- stand-up collar.
- over-blouses, 2-piece layered outfits.
- unbelted, high waistlines under the bust, also known as empire silhouettes.
- narrow belts sitting low on normal waistline.
- garments with waistband slightly below your normal waist, hip huggers.
- fabrics and designs unbroken from shoulder to hem when possible.

SHOULD AVOID

- waistlines that are high or built-up.
- wide belts.
- skirts that are box-pleated or gathered.
- garments that are thick and layered through the middle—this accentuates the small expanse between bust and hips.

3. BROAD HIPS, NARROW SHOULDERS

CAN WEAR

- collars extended past the shoulder line.
- soft shoulder pads.
- loose blouse not form-fitting.
- shawls.
- top sleeve seam with gathers.
- A-line skirts.
- darker colors on lower part of the body, lighter on top.
- vertical designs on fabrics.
- verticals on garments for the lower half of the body.

SHOULD AVOID

- shoulder seams of sleeves set in toward the neck.

- vests or sleeveless jackets that are wider at waist than at neck.
- gathered and box-pleated skirts.
- horizontal designs on lower half of body.
- fabrics that are bulky on hips.
- hip or patch pockets on any garments worn on lower part of the body.

4. NARROW HIPS, BROAD SHOULDERS

CAN WEAR

- full hair.
- V-neck tops to cut the width of the shoulders.
- front-button-down tops.
- single-breasted jackets.
- gathered or pleated skirts and dresses.
- darker colors on top part of the body, lighter on lower part.
- vertical and diagonal fabric designs on the torso.
- horizontal fabric designs around hips.
- pockets on skirts, pants and dresses at hip line.

SHOULD AVOID

- the "pinhead" look (pulled-back, flat hair).
- dress or blouse designs with yokes, collars or lapels that give a horizontal feeling.
- jackets or coats with padding in shoulders.
- double-breasted jackets.
- tailored suits.
- tight/snug pants.
- horizontal fabric designs on the lower part of body.

5. SMALL HIPS, LARGE CHEST

CAN WEAR

- special bra to help give rounded support instead of the "up" and "out" look.

- jewelry above bust.
- vests or sleeveless boleros (soft fabric).
- single-breasted jackets.
- softly detailed upper garments.
- dresses and skirts with flared effects that begin at waistline (pleats, gathers).
- darker-toned blouses and lighter-toned skirts or pants.

SHOULD AVOID

- high, round necks.
- frills, big scarves, bows, and other trimming near bust.
- tight, clinging sweaters, dresses and blouses.
- white or light colors on top.
- tight, exaggerated waistlines.
- wide belts.

6. SMALL CHEST, LARGE HIPS

CAN WEAR

- lined bra.
- full, feminine blouses.
- tops with shirring, tucks or pleats.
- vests or boleros.
- the "layered look" on top part of body (blouse with loose sweater or vest on top, left open).
- light-colored top with dark-colored bottom.
- emphasis on vertical designs in front-center of dress or skirt.
- skirts flaring gently from hips down.
- pantsuits with tunic or medium- to long-length jackets.

SHOULD AVOID

- tight-fitting, clingy blouses or sweaters.
- tailored blouses.
- gathered or box-pleated skirts and dresses.

- waistbands that are tight or exaggerated.
- short skirts above the knee, which tend to accentuate the hips.
- light-colored skirts or slacks.
- horizontal designs around hips.

TIPS FOR SPECIAL OCCASIONS:
NECK, SHOULDERS, STOMACH, THIGHS

NECK TOO LONG OR TOO THIN

CAN WEAR

- hair close to shoulder length (or longer if you wish).
- high necklines to break the long vertical line of the neck.
- fussy high necklines such as with big bows, ornate collars, ruffles.
- high scoop necklines with delicate jewelry.
- scarves or jewelry if you have a V-cut garment.

SHOULD AVOID

- upsweep or very short hairstyles. If you do wear your hair in an upsweep, be sure to break your neckline by wearing high collars, turtlenecks, high ruffles or jewelry .
- deep V-neckline.
- garments that leave the whole length of the neck and upper chest exposed.

NECK SHORT OR PLUMP

CAN WEAR

- hair up or away from your neck.
- simple necklines—the simpler the better.
- V-neck garments.
- low necklines.

Should avoid

- hairstyles that will cover up all of neck.
- anything fussy at the neck.
- high-neck styles.
- scarves.
- jewelry sitting on the neck itself (wear drop jewelry away from neck).

Shoulders Too Wide

Can wear

- tailored, smooth garments.
- seams slightly inside actual edge of shoulder line.
- closely fitted upper garments with vertical seams set in from each side.
- raglan sleeves (and other styles that "break" the shoulder line).
- fabrics with vertical designs.
- dark colors on upper half of body.

Should avoid

- shoulder pads.
- any gathering at shoulders, such as puffy sleeves.
- tight and clingy tops.
- double-breasted styles.
- garments that are too large for you.
- fabrics with horizontal lines.

Shoulders Too Narrow

Can wear

- soft shoulder pads, wide collars.
- extended shoulder line, crosswise yokes.
- shoulder seams on the outside of the shoulder.
- puffy and fussy sleeves.

- short, cap or puff sleeves.
- horizontal lines on garments.

SHOULD AVOID

- tight, clingy garments on upper half of the body.
- vests, boleros, or any other garment that would focus the attention on the center of the body.
- kimono and raglan sleeves.
- vertical fabric design.

STOMACH TOO LARGE

CAN WEAR

- the proper control undergarment.
- over-blouses, tunic-style tops that are loose, but not overflowing.
- narrow and loose belts (do not pull in too tightly as your stomach will appear fuller).
- garments that fit loosely across the stomach; if they are too tight, the stomach tends to be exaggerated.
- A-line, princess styles, darker color skirts and pants.
- flared skirts.
- darts in front of garments, over stomach, to make a smooth line at the waist.
- flat front, side or back zippers are best, if possible.

SHOULD AVOID

- empire styles.
- tight waistband styles of dress or top.
- wide or tight belts.
- garments that are too loose and flowing across the stomach, such as gathered skirts.
- garments that fit tightly under the stomach.
- gored skirts.

- thick fabric.
- front zippers.
- tight slacks; hip huggers.
- pants styles with trim or decoration (including belt loops, etc.) at the waist or over the stomach.

Thigh Bulges or Hips Too Large

Can wear

- jackets that come to the top of the largest area of the bulge.
- slightly flared skirts, A-line.
- slight pleat or draping effect.
- full-cut leg styles of slacks.
- full pedal pushers, knickers, culottes, gauchos, with a slight fullness.
- dark lower garments.
- vertical lines in fabrics on lower garments.
- medium to lightweight fabrics that do not cling.

Should avoid

- short skirts.
- straight or clingy skirts or slacks.
- tight-fitting pants.
- pockets or decoration around the thigh area.
- light colors on lower garments.

Waist Too Large

Can wear

- soft over-blouse or sweater.
- jackets that extend to hips.
- soft slim belt that ties.
- a waist cincher for a dress or outfit.

- fabrics that fall gracefully from waist—not too tight or baggy.
- solid medium-to-dark colors.

Should avoid

- wide belts or waistbands.
- high waistband or tight, wide midriff-band dress styles.
- gathered or pleated skirts.
- large, bright prints.
- pockets, belt loops, and other decorative trim at the waist.

Lose 10 Pounds in 10 Minutes

You have a special occasion coming up in a few days and you haven't lost those 10 pounds, yet want to look your best. Don't worry—I've got you covered!

There are 2 basic rules: one is to gain as much height as possible (in good taste) and the other is to "remove" the heaviest parts (width) of your body. You will need your full-length mirror—stand far enough away from it so that you can see your entire body from head to toe.

Should wear

- a hairstyle that gives a little height. But don't go overboard with your hair up or you will appear "head heavy," the balance will be wrong. Even if you wear your hair down and just combed out, you can puff the top a bit with subtle teasing.
- figure control panty hose.
- V-necklines—they lengthen the face and neck and give the illusion of greater slenderness and height in general.
- clothes that hug the largest part of your hips or body (but not tightly) such as A-line or slim line skirts and dresses with a slight flare at the bottom. Wear blouses that do not have excess material on the sides or above the waist area.
- smooth lines from shoulder to hem, simple and uncluttered long, narrow lapels on blouses, jackets and coats (this makes the wearer seem taller).

- hemlines that fall just below the knee or almost to the floor.
- soft fabrics such as silks, jerseys, soft cottons, soft lightweight synthetics.
- vertically designed fabrics from shoulder to hem. Stay with medium- or small-size fabric designs when not able to use a vertical design. Solids are good too.
- dark- to medium-color fabrics.
- medium to dark natural-tone stockings.
- high-heel shoes, but if you're wearing a long skirt, dress or pants they should be long enough to barely touch the top of shoe and cover most of the heel.

SHOULD AVOID

- flat hairstyles.
- turtlenecks—they cut length of neck and make body seem bulkier.
- double-breasted or wide lapels—adds width and decreases height.
- hems above the knee—the longer and more continuous the flow of a skirt or dress, the more height it gives you. (But hems should be no longer than 2 inches below the knee, unless they are floor length.)
- no excess material at the bottom of the blouse. Tucking too much extra fabric into the skirt adds width to the hips.
- accessories such as wide belts and sashes; they tend to cut into your height.
- "tent" styles.
- rough-textured fabrics such as tweed or heavy wools.
- horizontal stripes, large patterns, plaids, gathers, pleats, and large patch pockets—all these give width to hips and bust.
- wearing white or light solid colors—this adds more width to figure.
- flat shoes.

AFTERTHOUGHTS

OK, you've come this far, so I'll tell you...I guess you deserve to know: One flaw I have that nobody knows or notices—except maybe my husband, and I know he doesn't care—I have skinny legs. You'll hardly ever see me in a short skirt. I have a closet full of long skirts of every style and description, but no short skirts, and a collection of slacks and pants suits that I can wear anywhere. And I can easily direct the eye to those areas that are great, not only by using some of the techniques I've described, but also—and this is important for you to remember—by the manner and poise with which I carry myself. Throughout my career as a Wilhelmina model in New York City, not one photographer ever commented or complained about my skinny legs.

Did the illusion I created of having a great pair of gams succeed and become a reality? It certainly did!

PLASTIC SURGERY AND OTHER ENHANCEMENTS

Nobody thinks they are perfect...
even if they pretend they are!

If you have waited too long to get the results you would like, or are up in years and need a little extra help, don't give up. Here is a list for you to check out of treatments or procedures, types of professional and medical skin treatments, and plastic surgery.

Although I have not had a facelift myself—I had my eyes done in my late 30s, and I've had botox and collagen injections—I am not opposed to plastic surgery.

I believe there are 6 major reasons why I have not needed a facelift.

- My excellent bone density—my facial skull has not shrunk and neither has my body.

- I have not gained weight, adding extra fatty tissue to my facial surface.

- I have treated my skin with creams and lotions all my life and protected it from the sun's harmful rays.

- I also stimulated the collagen in my skin every day with my "Mini Facelift" cleansing routine.

- I have been on Hormone Replacement Therapy supervised by my doctor.

- I have never smoked.

But believe me, if I thought I needed a facelift, I'd wait in line to get one!

Non-surgical Treatments

Botox

Botox injection is a cosmetic procedure used to reduce fine lines and wrinkles. Small, diluted amounts can be injected directly into specific muscles, causing controlled weakening of the muscles. As a result, the injected muscle cannot contract, causing the wrinkles to relax and soften. Botox is most often used on forehead lines, crow's-feet around the eyes and frown lines. It generally takes about 5 days or more to take full effect. A small percentage of people may develop eyelid drooping, which usually resolves itself in 2 or 3 weeks. Not rubbing the treated area for 12 hours or laying down for 3 or 4 hours after the injection will help prevent drooping eyelids.

Collagen Injectable Fillers

Injectable fillers have become a popular facial rejuvenation treatment. As we age, the underlying tissues that keep our skin looking youthful and firm begin to break down due to the effects of gravity, sun exposure, diet, genetic factors and years of facial muscle movement. These factors over time contribute to the development of lines, wrinkles and folds in the face. Collagen injectable fillers give your skin a plumper and smoother look. Although collagen is the best-known filler, there are other substances that can be used, including fat from your own body and synthetic materials.

Types of fillers

- Zyderm and Zyplast are bovine-derived collagen products that replace the collagen your skin loses over time. They are placed just beneath the skin, in the dermis where the body accepts it as its own.

- CosmoDerm and CosmoPlast are bioengineered human collagen products that are used for similar indications as Zyderm and Zyplast, but have the advantage of not needing a skin test prior to the first treatment.

- Juvederm is an injectable gel approved by the FDA to last up to a year. It's especially good for the correction of moderate to severe facial wrinkles and folds.

- Artecoll is a synthetic filler, and because it's synthetic you are at higher risk of an allergic reaction, but it lasts much longer. You should have a skin test.

- Autologen is an injection of your own collagen. It's extracted from another place on your body. There's no risk of allergic reaction but the results are only temporary.

- Restylane is a clear gel. It contains hyaluronic acid, which naturally occurs in humans, so there's little chance for an allergic reaction. It's biodegradable, so your body will absorb it within about 6 months of the injection.

CHEMICAL PEELS

Also known as derma peeling, a chemical peel is a technique in which a chemical solution is applied to the skin. The treated skin peels off, leaving the new skin smoother. Chemical peels can be used on the face, neck or hands. They can help reduce wrinkles, sun spots, mild scarring, certain types of acne, freckles and age spots. After the chemical peel, your skin will be red. It will continue to peel for up to a week before the benefits can be seen.

DERMABRASION

Dermabrasion is an abrasive procedure that "sandblasts" the skin to create a smoother layer of skin. It is used to treat age spots, scars, pox marks and skin lesions. To perform the abrasion, the doctor uses a high-speed instrument equipped with a wheel or brush to strip off the top layers of skin. The risks can include uneven changes in skin color, scarring and infection.

LASER SKIN RESURFACING

In this procedure, the areas to be treated are numbed with a local anesthetic. A special dressing is applied to the treatment areas for about 24 hours. The healing process usually takes about 10 to 21 days, depending on where and how much was treated. Talk to your doctor about the possible reactivation of herpes cold sores and the need for an antibiotic if you have had herpes simplex cold sores in the past.

Laser Tattoo Removal

Lasers remove tattoos by breaking up the pigment colors with a high-intensity light beam and may take 2 to 4 treatments or more. The doctor activates a laser light which can be uncomfortable. An ice pack is applied to soothe the treated area. At each treatment, the tattoo should become a little lighter. A topical antibiotic cream or ointment should be used as a follow-up to protect the area. You must follow the doctor's instructions carefully in order to prevent possible infection and scarring.

Photodynamic Therapy

Photodynamic therapy is known for treating acne and sun damaged skin as well as for treatment of actinic keratosis, a precancerous skin lesion. The doctor applies a drug called a photosensitizing agent to the skin, in liquid form, and then exposes the area to a light that activates the agent and kills the lesion's cells. Side effects could be increased sensitivity to light, burns and swelling.

Vascular Laser Treatments

Lasers are used to treat spider veins, which are abnormal blood vessels on the face and head, and port-wine stains which are purple lesions on the face and neck. This is done by shrinking the dilated blood vessels. This treatment can be performed without anesthesia and usually must be repeated several times for complete results.

Plastic Surgery

Eyelid Surgery

Also known as blepharoplasty, eyelid surgery improves the appearance of the upper eyelids, lower eyelids, or both, and gives a rejuvenated appearance to the surrounding area of your eyes.

Brow Lift

Also known as a forehead lift, a brow lift minimizes the creases that develop across the forehead, or those that occur high on the bridge of the nose. It also improves what are commonly referred to as frown lines, and repositions a low or sagging brow.

FACELIFT

Also known as rhytidectomy, a facelift is a surgical procedure to improve visible signs of aging in the face and neck. It helps return the facial skin, muscle and underlying tissues to a more youthful contour. It will not stop the aging process but will offset some of its effects. The texture of your skin will not be modified. Skin conditions such as wrinkles, acne scars, age spots or smoker's creases around the lips will eventually return. There are many facelift choices which you can discuss with your surgeon.

LIPOSUCTION

Liposuction is a cosmetic surgical procedure that removes excess fat from underneath the skin. It can be used to get rid of saddlebags and love handles, and to sculpt areas such as the upper arms, calves, knee area, the outer breast area and back. Liposuction is not a weight procedure. It is known to remove stubborn areas of fat that have not responded to exercise and weight loss.

BREAST AUGMENTATION / BREAST IMPLANTS

Breast augmentation with implants is a cosmetic surgical procedure designed to either enlarge the breasts or to create symmetry if one breast is noticeably different in size and shape from the other.

Breast reduction (reduction mammaplasty) is a procedure designed to reduce the size of the breasts by removing fat, tissue and skin. It's often done by women who seek relief from pain in the back, neck and shoulders.

HOW TO CHOOSE A SURGEON

How do you choose a plastic surgeon you can trust, or any surgeon for that matter? Make sure the doctor is affiliated with a local hospital. If he is affiliated, he will be proud to tell you which one; if he is not, you'll want to run away as fast as you can! You can also call a hospital and ask for a recommendation for a surgeon. If affiliated, the hospital has scrutinized the background of the doctor for the safety of the hospital. The doctor does not have to have an office in the hospital, just be affiliated with it.

Be sure to choose a doctor who has been certified in his or her particular field of plastic surgery.

American Board of Surgeons (ABS)

The ABS certifies surgeons in the fields of general surgery, vascular surgery, pediatric surgery, surgical critical care, surgery of the hand, and hospice and palliative medicine. They are not certified for plastic surgery.

American Society of Plastic Surgery (ASPS)

Whether you're considering cosmetic or reconstructive plastic surgery, you want the skill of an ASPS member surgeon—a doctor with more than 6 years of surgical training and experience, with at least 3 years specifically in plastic surgery. Their training and experience make them more qualified to perform your cosmetic or reconstructive procedure.

The American Board of Facial Plastic and Reconstructive Surgery (ABPS) certifies surgeons exclusively in facial plastic and reconstructive surgery.

Afterthoughts

At my age, I don't blame people for thinking I've had a facelift. But when they ask me—and, yes, they really do ask me right to my face—I tell them I will not answer that question because, "You won't believe me so you must look for yourself," as I pull my hair back and present my face and ears for a close-up view. I do the same thing for the TV cameras. "Look for yourself," I say. If you run into me somewhere along the way, I'll let you take a look, too!

CHAPTER 16

GLAMOUR AT EVERY AGE

Get ready to dazzle.

Are some beautiful people really beautiful, or are they just glamorous? I say most of the time you can't really tell! Glamour is not based on a certain kind of face or body type. Yet, real glamour is dazzling…and mysterious…and beautiful, all at the same time!

The good news is: Every one of us can be glamorous and can command that kind of attention. It's not something you're born with. It's something you learn!

As I said earlier, it's not expensive clothing, jewelry or the latest hairstyle. Glamour is projected by a multitude of things that create an overall image of exceedingly good looks. It's not only obvious external manifestation, such as a nicely made-up face and well-groomed hair. It also includes poise, good manners, a certain glow, excellent posture, looking aware and alive, and showing an interest in other people.

So how do you get it? By paying attention to all details from head to toe, as well as developing a positive attitude toward life.

GLAMOUR CHECKLIST

Some of these suggestions I have already mentioned, but they bear repeating!

ACCESSORIES

Don't overdo the jewelry. So many people wear too much jewelry at one time: several bracelets, a couple of rings, and a necklace or 2, or even 3. It doesn't matter whether it's real or expensive, or just costume jewelry. Too much of it will make you look "junked up," and therefore unglamorous. I have been told that maybe I wear too little jewelry, and my reply is, "I don't want to wear more, *I* want to be the jewel." If you find yourself wondering whether or not you're wearing too much, take something off!

CLOTHING

No matter how fashionable any single component of your outfit might be, it is the whole "you" that must look great. A woman can be wearing the most expensive jewelry, have a gorgeous hairstyle, and the most up-to-date designer clothes, and each one of these things individually could be very striking indeed, but if they don't mix well, if they are incongruous, the overall image will be ruined and even become unflattering. If you want to turn heads, keep things looking uncluttered and simple. Remember your full-length mirror.

Don't forget to look at the back side of the outfit, too, in order to see how you look walking away. That's when many people check you out. A garment that's stained or has buttons or hooks missing is unglamorous. Don't wear clothing that does not suit your body, even if it is the most fashion-forward-looking garment. And don't be taken in by fads or trends. Remember, classic styles are in vogue forever.

SHOES

Run-down shoes with worn heels or in need of polish are unglamorous. If you're wearing casual sandals, paying attention to your feet and toenails is important. A run in a stocking is very unglamorous, although we all unavoidably "get caught" every now and then.

HAIR

Needless to say, clean, healthy-looking hair in a neat style and a nice cut that flatters your face is a must.

Hands and Nails

Take a good look at your hands: Being glamorous does not necessarily mean having long, sculptured, painted nails. You may if you wish, of course, if that's your style and they're not too long. Rather, "glamour" involves clean and manicured nails, more or less even in length (yes, you can do it at home). They can be short with clear or colored polish, but most importantly, they must look "cared for."

Posture

In addition to stealing your glamour and beauty, it takes only a few years of poor posture to hamper your flexibility. It makes you look older, unhappy and tired, and it's the first step toward dowager's hump, double chin, potbelly and swayback. And that's just on the outside! Inside the body it can exacerbate varicose veins, pinched nerves and heart strain, and age your bones and organs.

To be glamorous, good posture is essential whether you're sitting or standing. Please pay particular attention to the following "how to" suggestions. If you put your body in alignment, things will begin to fall into place: flatter stomach, straighter back, buttocks more tucked in, and a longer neck. And you'll move more gracefully, too.

- Stand with feet a few inches apart, toes pointed straight ahead and arms hanging loosely at your sides.

- Distribute your weight evenly on both legs by pressing evenly on the balls of your feet. Tighten the muscles in the front of your thigh.

- Slowly draw the buttocks tightly together.

- Now, slowly stretch your spine upward while drawing your shoulder blades together. Take care not to lift your shoulders or tilt your chin.

- Start each day by putting your body in alignment this way, until good posture is natural to you. It's good to have a friend share this activity with you so you can check each other's form.

Once again, good posture will help you look more glamorous, feel more alive and, most of all, keep your body healthier for your lifetime.

MAKEUP

In Chapter 13, the No-Mistake Makeup School instructs how to apply makeup so that you can present yourself in the most glamorous way possible. Here I want to reiterate the essential points. If they seem a little redundant, please bear with me, because they are sooo important.

- Ditch the loud or iridescent makeup. You cannot look glamorous with overdone makeup or poor color choices. The most unflattering makeup is bright blue iridescent eye shadow. It's loud and there is nothing natural-looking or pretty about it. In fact, that's about all you see on the face, it's so overpowering.

- No oily-looking face. An oily face is for bedtime when you are treating your skin. During the day, it accentuates any lines or wrinkles. Powder down and you will see a softer, younger-looking face.

- Orange lipstick is not easy for most people to wear and still look glamorous. Be careful here. Make sure your lipstick has enough earth tone in it to balance the harshness of the orange.

- Do not overdo rouge. This is where you have to watch carefully because if, like me, you like or need the color, you're likely to put on too much. Before going out, check yourself in 2 different kinds of light, and ask someone else—your husband or a friend—to give you feedback, too.

- Never, ever draw a single line for an eyebrow. Very unglamorous! Use short, light, quick upward strokes for each "hair" to make the eyebrows more natural-looking.

- Treat your neck the way you treat your face when applying makeup: Consider it all one. Your neck should blend in with your face tones. From a distance it looks unglamorous to have the face one color and the neck another.

A GLAMOROUS VOICE

What has your voice got to do with glamour? A lot! In the early 1930s when "talkies" became all the rage, the careers of many silent movie stars were over because their voices were not in keeping with the images they had projected. The movie musical "Singing in the Rain" is a fun, wonderful look at that era and the difficulties actors with poor voices had to contend with.

You may not be a movie star, but the sound and quality of your voice is just as important. Your voice is actually a wind instrument. Your lungs provide air, your vocal cords are vibrators, and your throat and mouth act as a "horn." When everything is in harmony, the voice can be like music to the ear—soothing and persuasive. But, when it is "off-key," it's like an out-of-tune musical instrument.

Fortunately, we can change our voice and tone if we wish. When I was in my 20s, I heard my voice for the first time on a tape recording and realized I needed to lower it a little. So I did.

How To Acquire a Glamorous Voice

- **Make sure you don't speak too fast.** Fast talk sounds impersonal, and overbearing and not poised, therefore not glamorous.

- **Nasal tone of voice.** The main cause of a weak, nasal voice is tension in the muscles at the back of the tongue. "Talking through your nose" is usually caused by not opening your mouth wide enough when speaking, which forces the sound into your sinuses and through your nose. Train the muscles at the back of your tongue to relax. Test this by holding your hand in front of your mouth and nose, then feel the air as you blow it alternately through your mouth, then your nose. When speaking, the air should be coming through your mouth in order for it to be clear and crisp.

- **Mumbling or speaking in a monotone voice.** This has an easy solution. Stretch your mouth open as wide as you can and repeat the vowels, A E I O U. See how closed your mouth has been? Practice this and you will soon "hear" yourself when you mumble.

- **A piercing, high-pitched voice.** The body is sensitive to sound, and a high-pitched voice that penetrates annoys most people. A lower-pitched voice strokes the body and gets more attention because it is more pleasing and so much more relaxing to listen to.

  Tense throat muscles can cause an artificially high voice. If this pertains to you, don't try to force your voice lower; rather, coax it by relaxing those tense muscles. Take a few deep breaths and say, "I don't think it's going to snow."

Then lower your voice and say it again. Keep doing this until you reach a level you're comfortable with. Then practice this "low" tone until you are accustomed to it.

Here are some vocal qualities and behaviors that are unbecoming and definitely unglamorous. If you happen to have any of them, learn to change them.

- Speaking in a loud or piercing voice.

- Laughing loudly.

- Whispering. Some people speak so softly that everyone around them has to strain to hear them. This is not glamorous either. Check with others on whether you are projecting enough. What may sound perfectly normal to you inside your head may be too soft on the outside.

Working on your voice can be a fun project. Next time you go to the store, take a deep breath, and just for fun and practice, try out your new voice on a sales clerk. You may like it! Don't forget to use your new sound on the phone, too. Your voice really counts there as well.

ADDITIONAL TIPS

- **Chewing gum.** One of the most unglamorous things you can do is to chew gum in public. You will never see an important businessperson, politician or socially prominent individual chewing gum. One day when I was about 10 years old, I was chewing gum and my father told me I looked like a cow chewing its cud. After that, I took note of how some of my classmates looked while chewing gum. Daddy was right! I quit!

- **Picking teeth.** It is never acceptable to pick your teeth in public. I can't believe how many grown people I see doing it. Someone I knew thought it was OK because he had an expensive gold toothpick that he carried around with him. It wasn't until I showed him an etiquette book that he finally quit pulling out his toothpick in a restaurant.

- **Smiling.** A pleasant face projects an open, friendly and inviting personality and will attract others to you. Smile frequently.

AFTERTHOUGHTS

By now I hope you realize that a pretty face, or graceful legs, or a sexy figure are not the primary criteria of true beauty. Consider Barbra Streisand and her famous nose, who looked utterly glamorous in the movie *The Way We Were*, co-starring with Robert Redford.

So you don't need to look like Brooke Shields, Jamie Lee Curtis, Mariah Carey or Betty Grable, each of whom had their legs insured for millions of dollars. Just look at me with my skinny legs, and tell me I'm not glamorous despite them!

And I trust you'll agree with me that youthful good looks on their own are nowhere near as exciting as having glamour for a lifetime. While physical beauty tends to tarnish a bit in later years, once a woman has developed glamour, she rarely loses it. Sophia Loren, who is one month younger than I am, is a case in point.

So ladies, understand that my passion is not to challenge you to be simply beautiful and healthy, but to become glamorous as well, and show the world your true beauty.

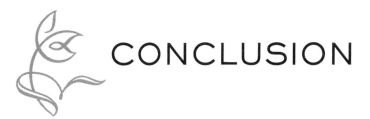

CONCLUSION

[People] do not quit playing because they grow old;
they grow old because they quit playing.

—Oliver Wendell Holmes

So many people actually speed up their aging process and then wonder how they got looking and feeling so old. Procrastination and lack of information are the two worst enemies of good health, beauty and youthfulness; and, as I mentioned earlier, the best anti-aging antidote is prevention. I learned this as a child from my father. He constantly preached prevention, mainly with regard to nutrition and diet; and I listened!

To keep optimally healthy and youthful, prevention has to cover everything—from your head to your toes, inside and outside. It's like taking care of your car. It operates best when all of its parts are running well and in sync. If you don't take care of it with regular maintenance, it won't run smoothly and is liable to shut down. It's the same with your body—it will not keep running on its own.

I believe more than half of my success has been due to the way I have tried to protect myself against potential problems in all aspects of my life, but especially in regard to my health, looks and longevity. And I'm not letting up. Indeed, at age 75, I'm intensifying it.

I don't care how old you are, it's never too late to start. It's never too early either. If you develop a mindset that focuses on "preventing," and practice it, you will enjoy a new sense of inner strength and self-esteem.

If you have absorbed the advice on these pages, you have conquered one enemy: lack of information. Keep the book handy as a reference, but don't stop there. Keep looking for answers, as I do. Advances in scientific development are made every day. Stay up on them. And please, avoid the pitfall of health and beauty's other worst enemy: procrastination.

No matter what new programs and products doctors and scientists invent for our good health, good looks and longevity, it will still be up to each one of us individually to implement them on a daily basis. No one else can do it for us and, as I have said before, there are no shortcuts.

> I WOULD RATHER TRY AND FAIL THAN WONDER WHAT MIGHT HAVE HAPPENED WHEN SITTING IN MY ROCKING CHAIR AT AGE 100.

Do we get old because we allow our bodies to slow down? That is a question each of us must answer for ourselves. By now you know my answer: We can't avoid getting older, but we don't have to look or feel like it.

I hope that my example will inspire you, and that what I have shared with you in these pages will allow you, too, to break the age barrier and enjoy good looks and health, whatever your age.

C'mon, get going. Come join me in my ageless world.

Love,
Oleda
Born 1934

 REFERENCES

Introduction

1. Hershkind, et al, "Human Genetics" 97: 319-23, The Danish Twin Study, 1996.

2. Butler, Robert N., M. D., "The Longevity Prescription, 8 Proven Keys to a Long, Healthy Life," Penguin Group (USA), May 2010.

Chapter 1

3. International Agency for Research on Cancer, The Lancet Oncology, World Health Organization, August 2009.

Chapter 3

4. Kerrigan, D.; Lelas, J.; Karyosky, M; "Women's Shoes and Knee Osteoarthritis," The Lancet, Volume 357, Issue 9262, Pages 1097-1098.

Chapter 6

5. U.S. Department of Health and Human Services, NIH News (National Institutes of Health), "NIHSeniorHealth.gov Offers Tips on Eating Well As You Get Older," May 2008.

Chapter 7

6. U.S. Department of Health and Human Services, Agency for Healthcare Research and Quality, "Postmenopausal Hormone Replacement Therapy for Primary Prevention of Chronic Conditions," 2004.

7. Cutler, Winnifred, PhD, "Hormones and Your Health," John Wiley & Sons, Inc., Hoboken, New Jersey, 2009.

8. British Medical Journal online, as reported in The Sunday Times (London), August 22, 2008.

9. Lobo, Rogerio A., M.D., Chairman, OB/GYN, Sloane Hospital for Women, NewYork-Presbyterian Hospital/Columbia University Medical Center, New York, NY, "Innovations in Hormone Replacement." Available at The Female Patient, www.femalepatient.com.

10. The Kronos Early Prevention Study, Kronos Longevity Research Institute. Available at www.keepstudy.org/keeps/why.cfm.

Chapter 8

11. U.S. Department of Health and Human Services, NIH News (National Institutes of Health), "Obesity Threatens to Cut U.S. Life Expectancy," March 2005.

12. U.S. Department of Health and Human Services, Office of the Surgeon General, "The Surgeon General's Call to Action," January 2007.

Chapter 9

13. Centers for Disease Control and Prevention, "Growing Stronger—Strength Training for Older Adults." Available at www.cdc.gov/physicalactivity/growingstronger/index.html.

Chapter 10

14. Eriksson, Peter S.; Perfilieva, Ekaterina; Björk-Eriksson, Thomas; Alborn, Ann-Marie; Nordborg, Claes; Peterson, Daniel A.; Gage, Fred H., "Neurogenesis in the Adult Human Hippocampus," Nature Medicine, November 1998.

15. Bakken, Rachel C.; Carey, James R.; De Fabio, Richard P.; Erlandson, Trevor J.; Hake, Jannifer I.; Intihar, Todd W.; "Effect of Aerobic Exercise on Tracking Performance in Elderly People: A Pilot Study," Journal of the American Physical Therapy Association, December 2001.

16. Cai, Denise J.; Mednick, Sarnoff A.; Harrison, Elizabeth M.; Kanady, Jennifer C.; Mednick, Sara C.; "REM, not incubation, improves creativity by priming associative networks," PNAS (Proceedings of the National Academy of Sciences), June 2009.

Chapter 11

17. Coren, Stanley, PhD, "Sleep Deprivation, Psychosis and Mental Efficiency," Psychiatric Times, March 1998.

18. Available at www.sleep-deprivation.com.

19. Neubauer, David N., M.D., "Sleep Problems in the Elderly," American Family Physician, May 1999.

INDEX

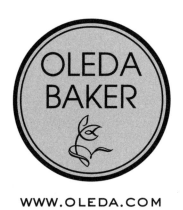

WWW.OLEDA.COM